A New Diagnostic Tool for Prolo Therapy
Structural Diagnostic Photography

by

James Carlson, D.O.

Copyright July 3, 2010

Published by The Arthritis Trust of America
7111 Sweetgum Road
Fairview, TN 37062

Edited by Anthony di Fabio

PREFACE

James Carlson, D.O. was one of the original Prolo Therapy pioneers.

It is with the greatest pleasure that we introduce you to Dr. James A. Carlson's novel and effective method for diagnosing structural problems[1]. After once determined, and if repairable, he normally solved these structural problems by known osteopathic procedures plus the judicious use of prolotherapy (also called proliferative therapy, sclerotherapy, or reconstructive therapy)[2].

The very first prolotherapy was probably performed by Roman soldiers who, in helping their wounded comrades, would place a hot spear point at a position which would assist in strengthening ligaments in such a way that a dislocated shoulder would recover.

Of course, modern treatments are not quite so harsh, as much has been learned about strengthening ligaments..

Although there are perhaps more than 1000 prolotherapists in the United States — MDs and DOs who practice some form of prolo therapy — only 39 are fully certified sclerotherapists, according to the American Osteopathic Association. Each must study beyond their medical diploma, and only a small handful of these practitioners are really excellent.

James A. Carlson, D.O. was not just a pioneer but also one among the very best!

Dr. Carlson also uses "Intraneural Injections[3]" and "Neural Therapy[4]."

Specialists in musculoskeletal pain have long used area-wide, i.e., non-specific "trigger points," intraneural injections and intra-articular injections, as well as nerve blocks to relieve pain. (The term "trigger points" is not always used the same way in these various procedures by different practitioners.) In other words, although their medical territory was not really inclusive, they unwittingly discovered some of the same patient points for pain relief[5].

To summarize the important additional techniques used by Dr. Carlson to bring about rapid permanent pain relief in many of his patients, he uses:

1. Osteopathic methods
2. Standard medical tests, such as blood samples and so on.
3. Prolotherapy (also called proliferative therapy, sclero- therapy, reconstructive therapy)
4. Intraneural injections (or specific injection therapy, injection therapy)
5. Neural injections (trigger point therapy)

His knowledge of where to use these various techniques, of course, comes from years of study and a great deal of successful experience.

During a number of those years Dr. Carlson began testing out a diagnostic method that he checked and cross-checked with every standard modality until he was able to rely upon his new technique for indications of where to apply the various injection modalities for swift, effective structural correction.

During the era of multi-million dollar diagnostic medical devices — and the prestige that seems to come with owning and using such devices — Dr. Carlson's recommended equipment — believe it or not — consisted of the following:

1. A polaroid camera (with film). *Of course nowdays you can use your digital camera, download the pictures into your computer and print out an 8.5" X 11" copy for diagnostics.*
2. A plumbob (with string)
3. A straight edge (and pencil)
4. Compass (with pencil)

Oh yes, and you need an excellent knowledge of anatomy!

In addition to a formal osteopathic degree and experience, Dr. Carlson was a physical therapist and certified athletic trainer for 13 years all of which required a superb knowledge of anatomy!!

One of us (Anthony di Fabio) has personally witnessed Dr. Carlson's phenomenal success with patients. We also have known him for many years as a personable, intelligent, honest and reliable osteopathic medical practitioner.

What he has to offer in this booklet is important and will surely advance the art of healing!

Learn it, go forth, and do likewise!!

References

1. Dr. Carlson has deep appreciation and gives thanks for early help from Fred L. Mitchell, Jr., D.O., F.A.A.O., F.C.A., Professor Emeritus of Osteopathic Manipulative Medical College of Osteopathic Medicine, Michigan State University, East Lansing, Michigan. Especially he gives thanks to Dr. Mitchell for the sharing of important knowledge through three publications, each entitled *The Muscle Energy Manual*. Volume I (1995), Volume II (2002), and Volume III (1999) are available thru MET Press, East Lansing, MI.

2. It's widely known that prolotherapy was used on Charles Everett Koop, M.D. — the Surgeon General of the United States from 1982 to 1989 under Ronald Reagan's presidency — to solve his intransigent and painful back problem. He was so impressed he began using prolo therapy on his own patients.

3. The Arthritis Trust of America feels that the booklet, *Intraneural Injections* formly titled *Intraneural Injections for Rheumatoid Arthritis and Osteoarthritis & The Control of Pain in Arthritis of the Knee,* by Dr. Paul K. Pybus, is a must for all forms of arthritis and arthri- tis-like pain, and that the use where appropriate of designated intraneural injections decreases the time to wellness, regardless of what other modalities are used on the patient. One important advantage being the ability to get the patient off of damaging pain-relieving drugs while the body is adapting to healing treatments and wellness routines.

Englishman Roger Wyburn-Mason, M.D., Ph.D., nerve specialist, was the first to describe the source principle (not causation) of joint damage from tender nerve locations, sometimes called "trigger points," in arthritis and arthritis-like pain.

South African Dr. Paul K. Pybus, his former house physician, learned to implement in clinical practice Wyburn-Mason's theories of intraneural injections, successfully using his discoveries for more than 20 years.

Keith McElroy, M.D. (The New York Orthopaedic Hospital) independently discovered the same principles, and applied them to his patients, also for many years. He calls them "Injection Therapy."

Dr. Paul K. Pybus and Gus J. Prosch, Jr., M.D. explored additional key "trigger points," until it became clear to them that a virtual one-to-one correspondence existed between painful neuroma and acupuncture points — but not always so.

Dr. I.H.J. Bourne, a friend of both Roger Wyburn-Mason and Paul Pybus, also developed the use of intraneural injections which he published as "Mu4. Neural Therapy (Injections), developed by Ferdinand and Walter Huenke, also about 70 years ago, addresses the problem of patterns of stored "pain" reflexes which trigger off permanent relief upon injection. These injections are par- ticularly important when addressing scar tissue and the abil- ity of such permanent scars to distort structure.

4. Neural Therapy (Injections), developed by Ferdinand and Walter Huenke, also about 70 years ago, addresses the problem of patterns of stored "pain" reflexes which trigger off permanent relief upon injection. These injections are particularly important when addressing scar tissue and the ability of such permanent scars to distort structure.

5. Dr. Curt Maxwell of Los Algodones, Mexico uses all injection modalities. While not addressing itself to inflamed neuroma, he also recommends the W.B. Saunders book, *Atlas of Pain Management Injection Techniques* by Steven D. Waldman, M.D., J.D. as an excellent supplementary book. (It is very convenient for doctors who are into reimbursement via insurance, as it gives the insurance code that is acceptable for each of the injections.) The artwork is excellent, and there can be no doubt as to how to do their recommended injections in the various parts of the body, but also contraindications, et. al.

Anthony di Fabio. M.A.
Perry A. Chapdelaine, Jr. M.D., M.S.P.H.

INTRODUCTION

Since the advent of the profession of osteopathy in the late nineteenth century there has been an increasing recognition that the relationship of the compression members (bones) are regulated by the soft tissues. These soft tissues constitute muscle ligaments, joint capsules, intervertebral discs, synovial surfaces, and, very importantly, fascial sheets within the body.

Traditionally, the osteopathic lesion has been more recently replaced by the term somatic dysfunction. Terms such as *motion segments and alignment* have all been predicated on various techniques for defining the position of the skeletal system. Neglected in these systems has been a discussion of the governing tissues concerned; that is to say, nerves and muscles.

Many physical schools have focused on the function of somatic muscles, again frequently ignoring the role of the passive, yet critically important muscles, ligaments and fasciae.

The fascial tubes of the body, as well as the ligaments, define the motion, normal and abnormal, between the hard components, i.e., the compression members, the bones. As it is, there has grown in the last decade, or more, a gradual interest in defining these tension members, their properties both in health and after injuries, and possibly in diseased conditions. Some of the terms which are coming into use regarding the tension members include tensile-strength, elasticity, interactive relationships, hysteresis, and, most importantly, *tensegrity.*

A significant problem in defining the properties of the tension members is the difficulty in defining landmarks by an imaging technique, or, for that matter, by palpation. There are, however, certain areas of the tubular form of the human frame in which the soft tissues adhere more-or-less firmly to visible external landmarks. Varying tensions within the fascial tubes of the body, therefore, affect these parts. The head is separated from the trunk by the neck, which can be considered, for the purpose of this paper, as a narrow *funnel* through which the longitudinal fascial tensions pass. Strains placed on the human head due to distortions in the fascial tube of the trunk serve, it is found, as magnifiers and definers of these distortions. This is the simple basis of Structural Diagnostic Photography, or SDP. (In the practice of Structural Diagnostic Photography, the pelvis and the head are reciprocals of one another. The tubular body receives, accepts and stores energy via pulley and pulley wheels and levers and fulcrums. SDP is a simple method of determining those forces, and recommending methods for untangling them.)

Most distortions in the human fascial tube are due to dysfunctions in the pelvis.

The position of the head was thought, as a first approximation, to reflect fascial tensions transmitted from the body. Should there be significant distortion in the alignment of the endoskeleton (and the pelvis in particular) versus the fascial tube of the trunk, it is likely to be reflected in subtle changes in the position of the head through this transmission mechanism.

Can a photographic analysis of the position of the head -- versus the trunk -- reveal these distortions? If so, by what mechanism can a clinician take advantage of these observations?

The purpose of this paper is to evaluate such a system developed by the author in his private practice in Knoxville, Tennessee, over the course of the last decade of the twentieth century.

A series of linear markings is extended from specific defined points on the head upwards and over the trunk downwards. The patterns caused by these lines and their relationship to the midline of the trunk, defined with a plumb line while the patient stands, appear to yield information about what has hitherto been defined as somatic dysfunction of the axial skeleton. This scheme -- *Structural Diagnostic Photography* (SDP) -- parallels the diagnostic utility of manual techniques which have been traditional in the osteopathic profession. The effectiveness of this imaging technique has been validated internally in the study by assessing changes in the linear markings after treatment. Treatment sessions were based on standard osteopathic medicine routines, to wit: 1) osteopathic manipulation, 2) osteopathic medical techniques, and 3) cranial osteopathic techniques.

MATERIALS AND METHODS
Imaging Routine

The method involves taking a frontal Polaroid photo (or digiatal camera) of the subject and drawing certain lines on the photo (or a photocopy of the actual photograph). The relation of the lines implies a fascial symmetry or lack thereof. The photo is taken in a more-or-less (approximate) standardized format and includes the head and trunk at least to below the knees. A plumb-line hangs from the ceiling in front of the subject at a well-defined and always-used position, and the photographer centers the patient on the line, plumb-line in front of the body, back in front of the wall.

A photo is taken with a standard flash Polaroid type of camera (or modern digital camera) while the patient stands in front of a dark wall. Although the actual photo can be used, in my practice I preserve it without marks as a part of the patient's permanent record. A copy machine copy is made of the photo, or computer print out, and, using the copied image, the photograph is

Figure 1b

vectored with straight lines defined by points marked

on the image of the face. Then lines are drawn from these points of the face as shown in Figure 1b below:

A point from the medial corner of the eye to the lateral margin of the mouth on the same side are defined and a ruler placed through them. A line is then drawn (extended) with a pencil over the whole photograph and, if need be, extended across the background paper on which the copy of the photograph is made or pasted.

The second line is drawn from the side of the head and following the sternocleidmastoid muscle outline.

According to this method (Structural Diagnostic Photography) it is assumed that in optimal health (and body symmetry) the lines do not converge. In the patient population evaluated for this study convergence was observed to be variable and common.

The site of crossing of the "parallel lines" is noted in detail. It is assumed that such a convergence and its location represent fascial abnormalities which call for osteopathic treatment.

In selected patients, treatment includes foot taping, shoe lifts, and prolo therapy.

The convergence may be either inferior or superior. If the convergence is inferior there is a posterior dysfunction. If the convergence is superior it is an anterior dysfunction on the contralateral side.

If the lines converge below the head, usually somewhere over the lower trunk, groin or thigh area, there is a posterior dysfunction of the sacroiliac joint, with an ilium that is rotated posteriorly on the same side. (See Figure 8.) In these cases there is likely to be an abnormality of the anterior or posterior sacro-illiac joints.

If superior, convergence extends to the lumbar region, there is a lumbar plexus intervated structure present..

If onvergence is inferior and extends to the lower lumbar or pelvis, a sciatic plexus intervated structure is involved.

When there is a superior convergence of lines or lines above the head there is contra-lateral dysfunction which is anterior.

When there is an inferior convergence of lines or lines below the head there is contra-lateral dysfunction which is posterior.

If the lines converge above the head, with the use of a compass the arc can be brought around and falls within the pelvis, an anterior sacroiliac dysfunction on the contralateral side exists.

2

If the arc falls within the thorax, a costovertebrae dysfunction exists at the level of the arc. It would be an anterior dysfunction on the contralateral side.

Conversely, if the inferior convergence falls within the trunk it suggests a posterior dysfunction on the same side at that level.

The center prong of the compass, i.e., the one with a needle, is placed on the temporal nasion junction of the photo, the other end, i.e., the one with the pencil point is placed over the point of convergence. The compass is rotated over its sharp point and a half-circle drawn over the front of the body des

A fir
top of the
the whol
below th
the line
of the ea
photo.

Line
parallel.
the right
be referr
lines. Wl
that there
head (os
side of
Treatmer
palatine
the sphe
mobiliz
side.

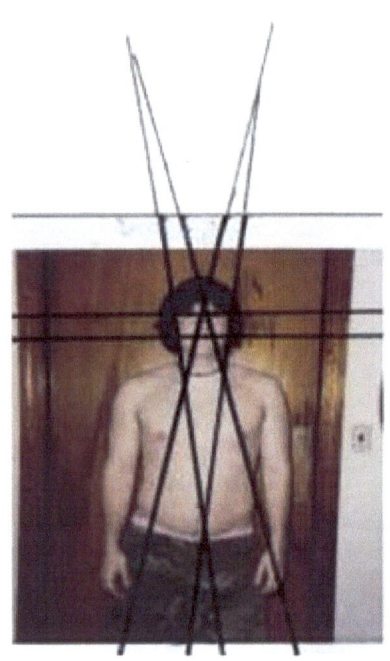

Figure 1a: Pre-treatment

Patients

Sixty patients' charts culled in sequence from a private osteopathic practice in Knoxville Tennessee between 1998 and 2001 constitute the patient population of this study. their individual styles. This comment regarding treatment modalities applies to this author's practice, as well.

The relationship of the analyzed observations before and after treatment are tabulated for all the subjects. The before and after figures on page 64 is a sample illustration of characteristic findings in a case before and after treatment. Cases were discarded from the study only on the basis of inadequate quality of images, or for attendances for problems other than musculoskeletal ones. That is to say that to the extent feasible in a private practice setting, any bias by exclusion of unsuitable subjects was avoided.

As indicated in Table 1, above, the osteopathic medical techniques used in treatment of these subjects *changed* the definition of fascial tubular alignment abnormalities in 78% of the cases. Based on the traditional osteopathic concept, an approximation to perfect symmetry represents an improvement in

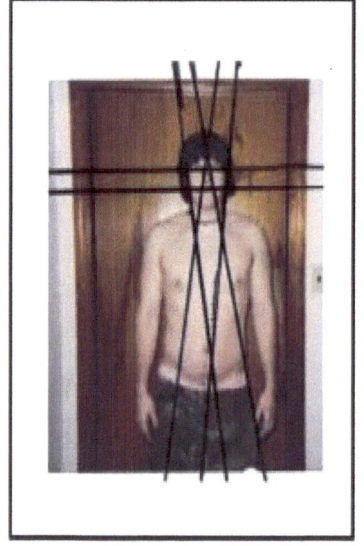

Figure 1b: Post-treatment
More Parallel

health. The treatment modalities have led to such an improvement in 80.5 % of cases. Review of the charts representing cases in which failure of

RESULTS					
Table I					
Patients Total	Craniel Component	Posterior	Anterior	Dorsal	Syphasis
60	18	19	37	11	14

improvement in the fascial lines as defined here for Structural Diagnostic Photography (SDP) disclosed that a defined and recognized cause could be identified. The causes included 1) imbalance in remaining wisdom teeth, 2) improperly tensed braces on teeth, 3) unsuitable dentures, 4) chronic contractures which included the fascial layers of the body, 5) cosmetic surgery, and 6) orthopedic sur- gical implants.

Conclusion

A new vision is introduced into osteopathy with this paper. A technique for defining abnormal fascial strain in the (tubular) human frame based on the multiplication effect of the distortion of these forces through the "funnel" of the neck on the head has been utilized to define a graphic method of cataloging these tensions, correlating them with traditional definitions of somatic dysfunction and evaluating treatment outcomes.

It is hoped that this new approach will focus future clinical researchers on the importance of the soft tissues in regulating form and function in the human frame, and facilitate a better understanding and definition of these tissues. After all, the alignment of the bones is secondary to abnormalities in tension of the soft tissues or vice versa.

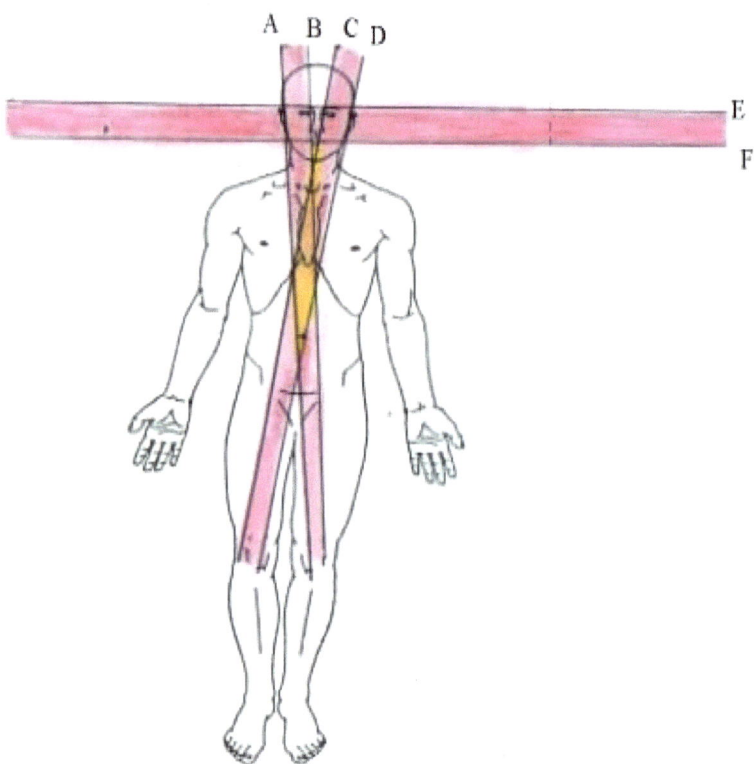

Figure 1. Normal

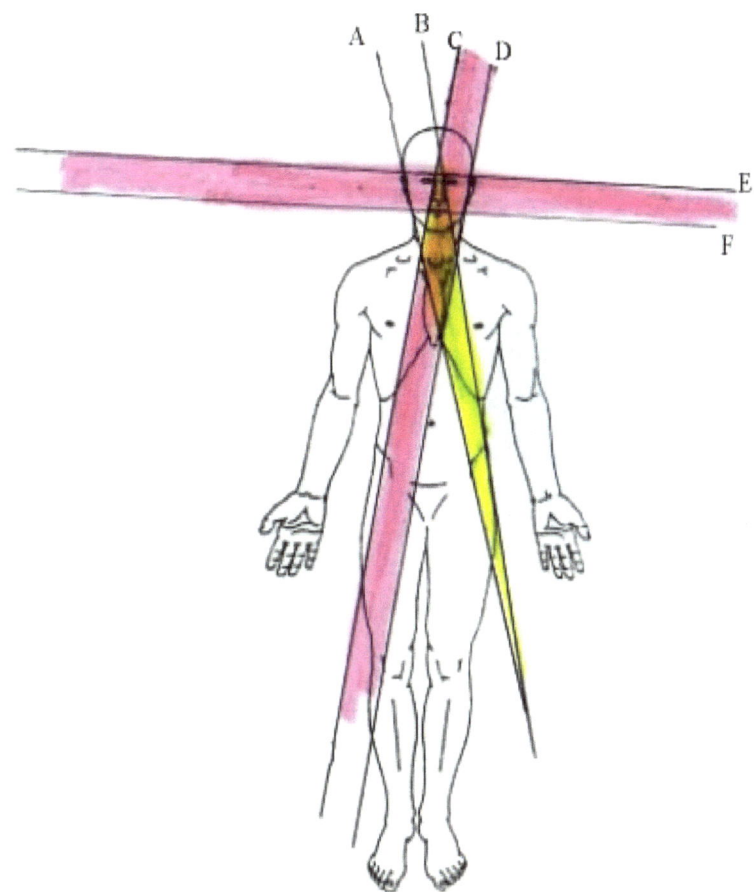

FIGURE 2.

This is much like the pattern in Figure 8. It shows an internally rotated pattern but with the inferolateral convergence being outside the lower legs. This usually indicates that one of the symptoms the patient will have is dizziness. This pattern is seen most often in the elderly.

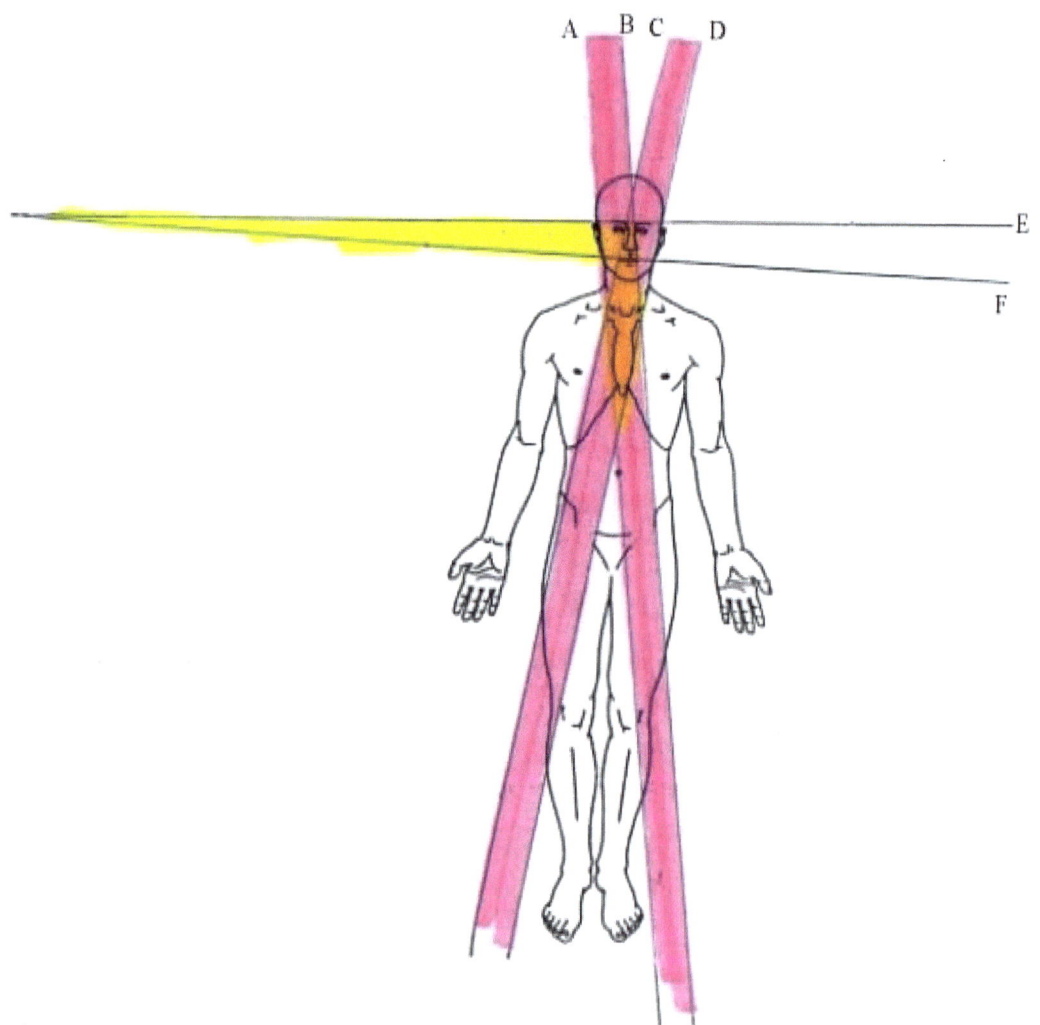

A B C D

—E

F

FIGURE 3.

This can come from either side ond represents
a side bending crainial strain.

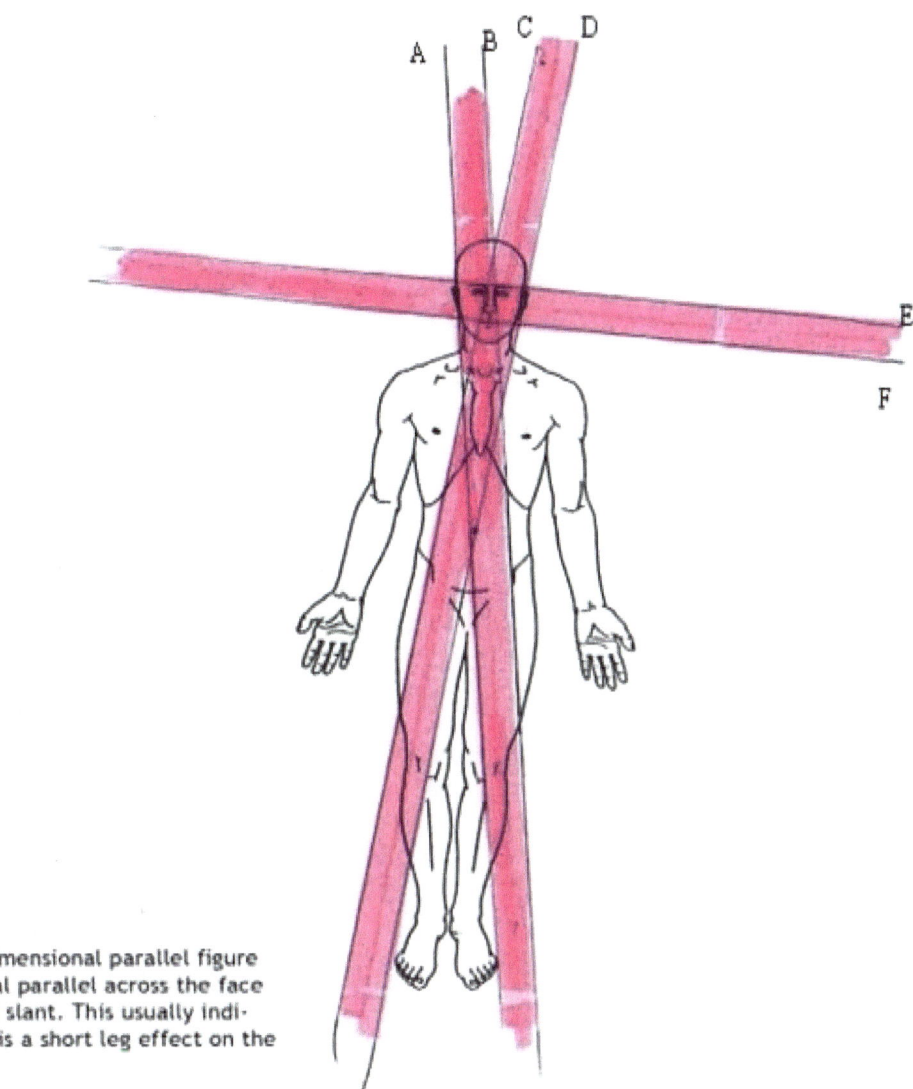

FIGURE 4.

This shows a 3 dimensional parallel figure but the horizontal parallel across the face shows a downard slant. This usually indicates that there is a short leg effect on the inferior side.

8

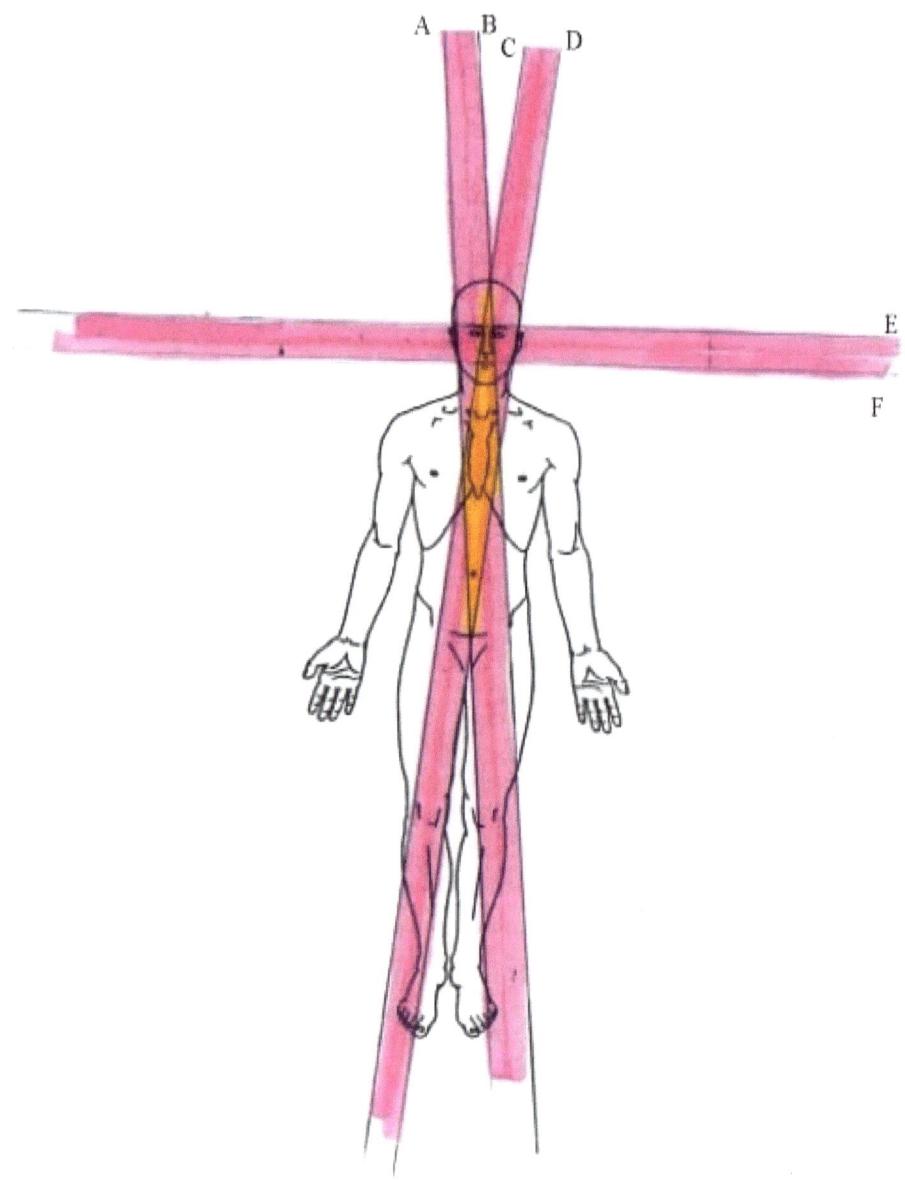

Figure 5

This pattern shows lines A & D converging on the pubic symphysis indicating a pubic symphysis involvement either ligamentous or from a degenerative symphysial disk allowing spurring and arthritic rubbing. This is also seen at times with people with involved prostates or bladder involvement.

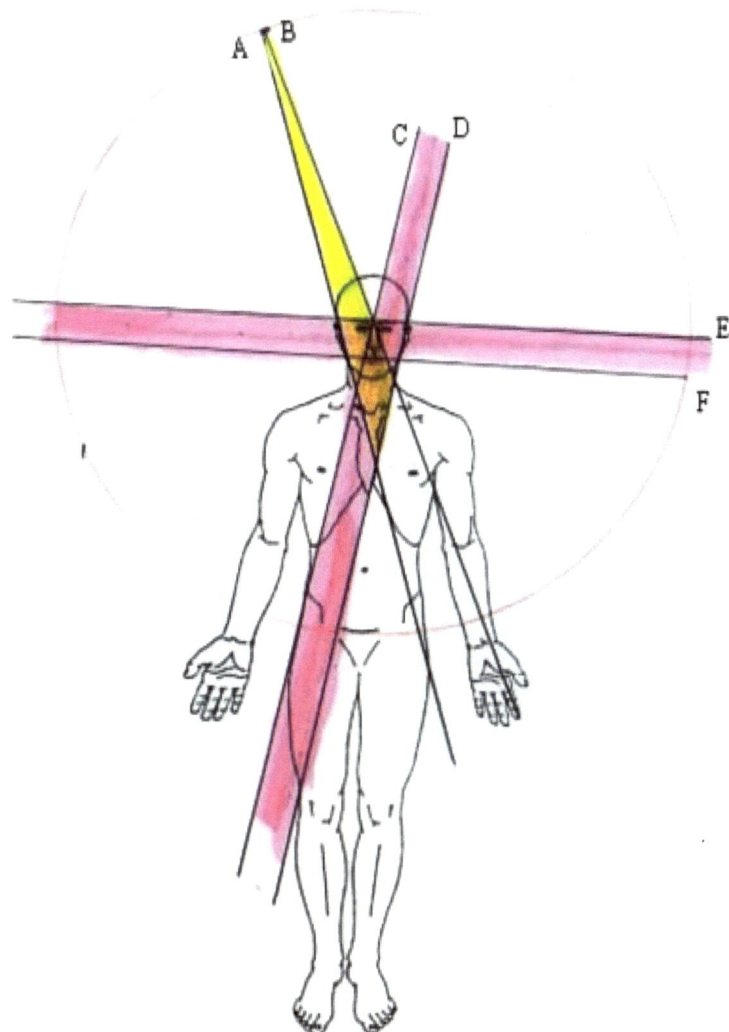

FIGURE 6.

This pattern depicts a convergence of lines above the head which indicates an anterior strain pattern on the contralateral side. Place the center of the compass between the eyes and strike an arc thru the convergence. In this particular case, it would indicate an anterior sacroiliac involvement.

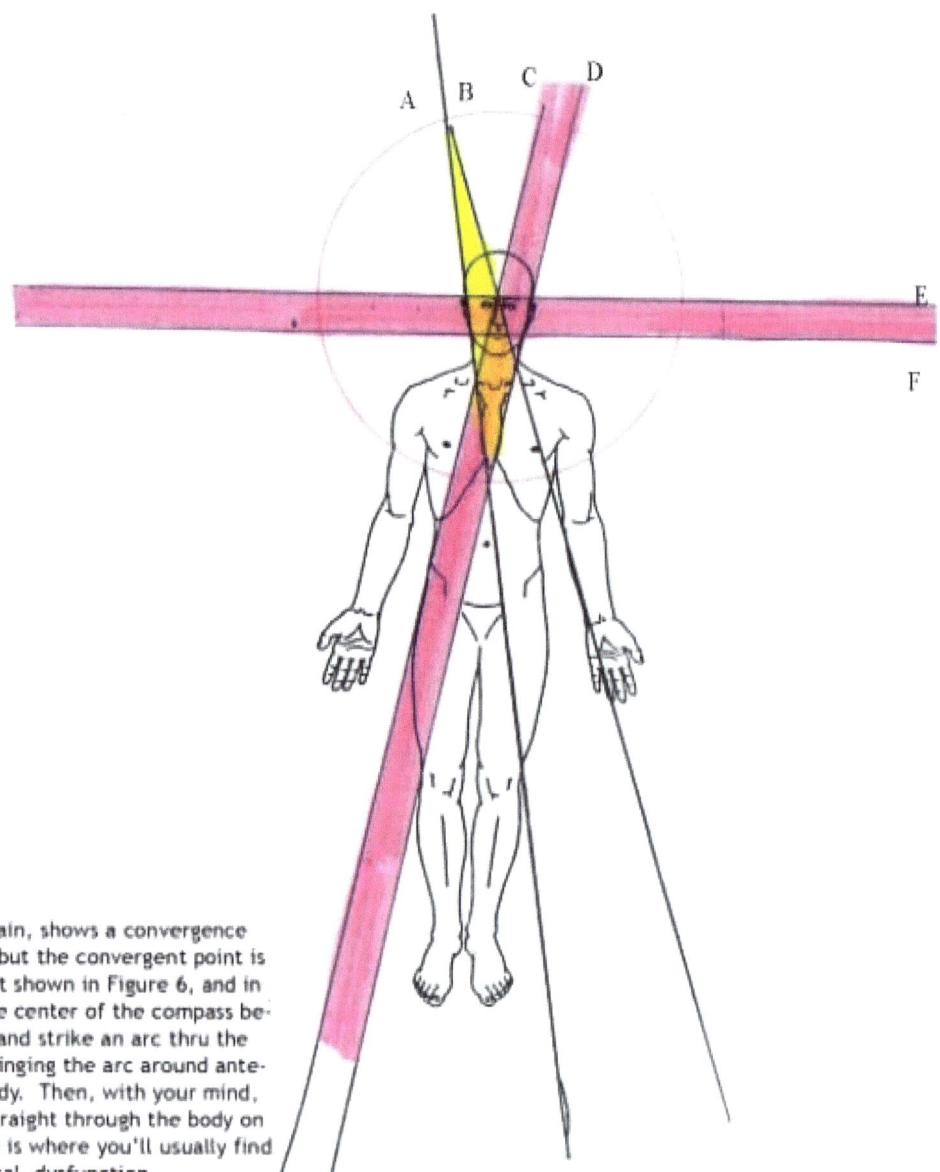

FIGURE 7.

This pattern, again, shows a convergence above the head but the convergent point is shorter than that shown in Figure 6, and in this case, set the center of the compass between the eyes and strike an arc thru the convergence, bringing the arc around anteriorly on the body. Then, with your mind, locate a point straight through the body on the spine. There is where you'll usually find vertebral or costal dysfunction.

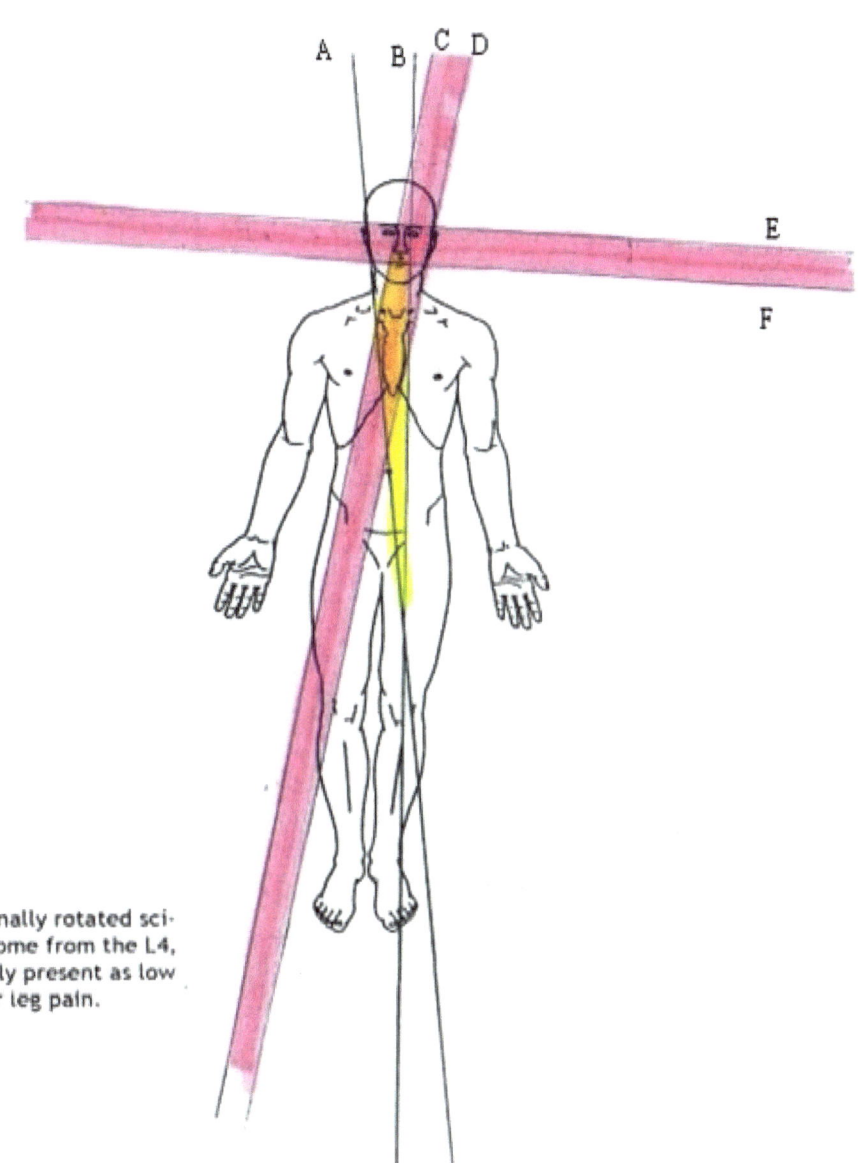

FIGURE 8.

This pattern is an internally rotated sciatic pattern that can come from the L4, L5, S1, and will probably present as low back pain and posterior leg pain.

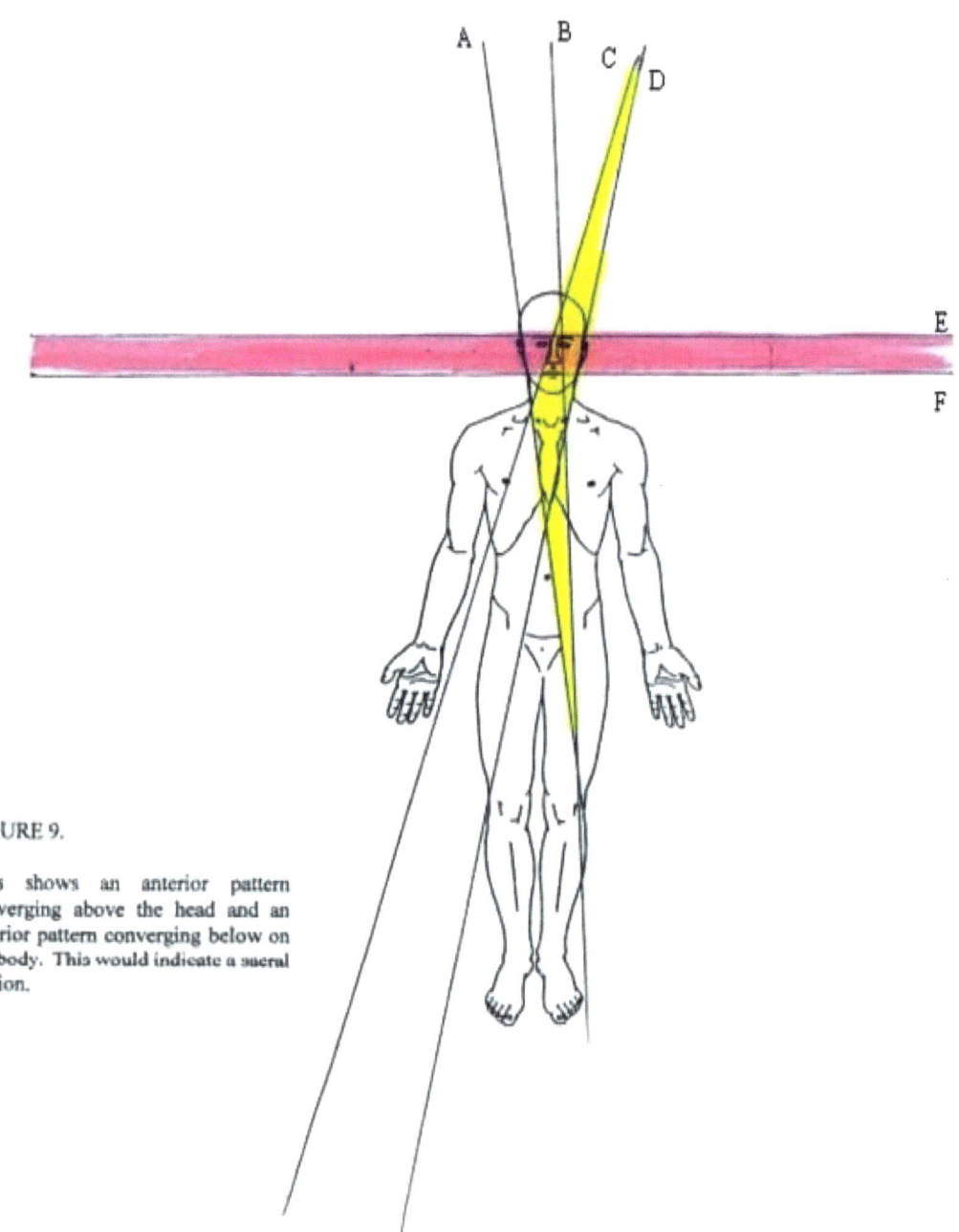

FIGURE 9.

This shows an anterior pattern converging above the head and an inferior pattern converging below on the body. This would indicate a sacral torsion.

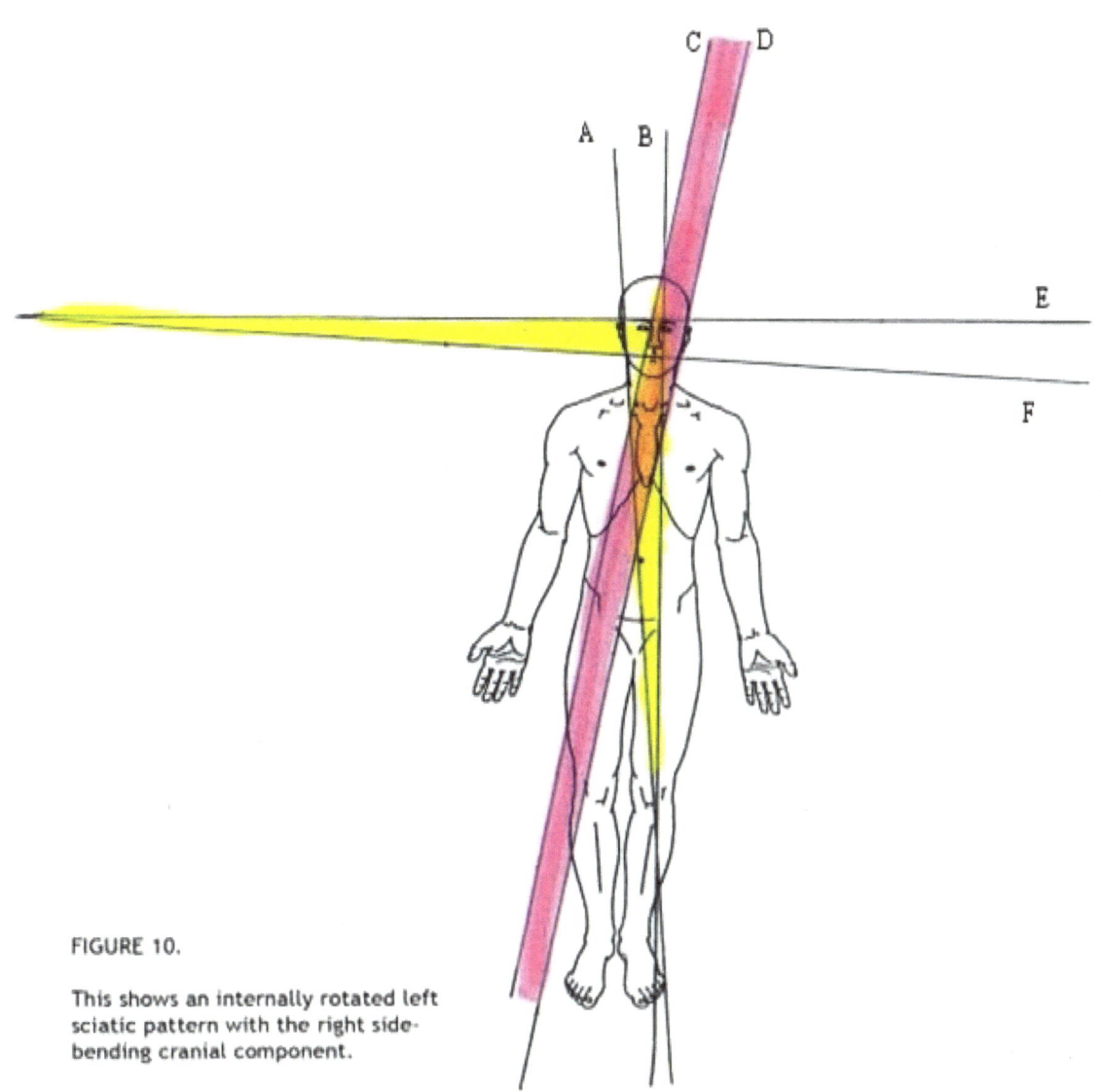

FIGURE 10.

This shows an internally rotated left sciatic pattern with the right side-bending cranial component.

14

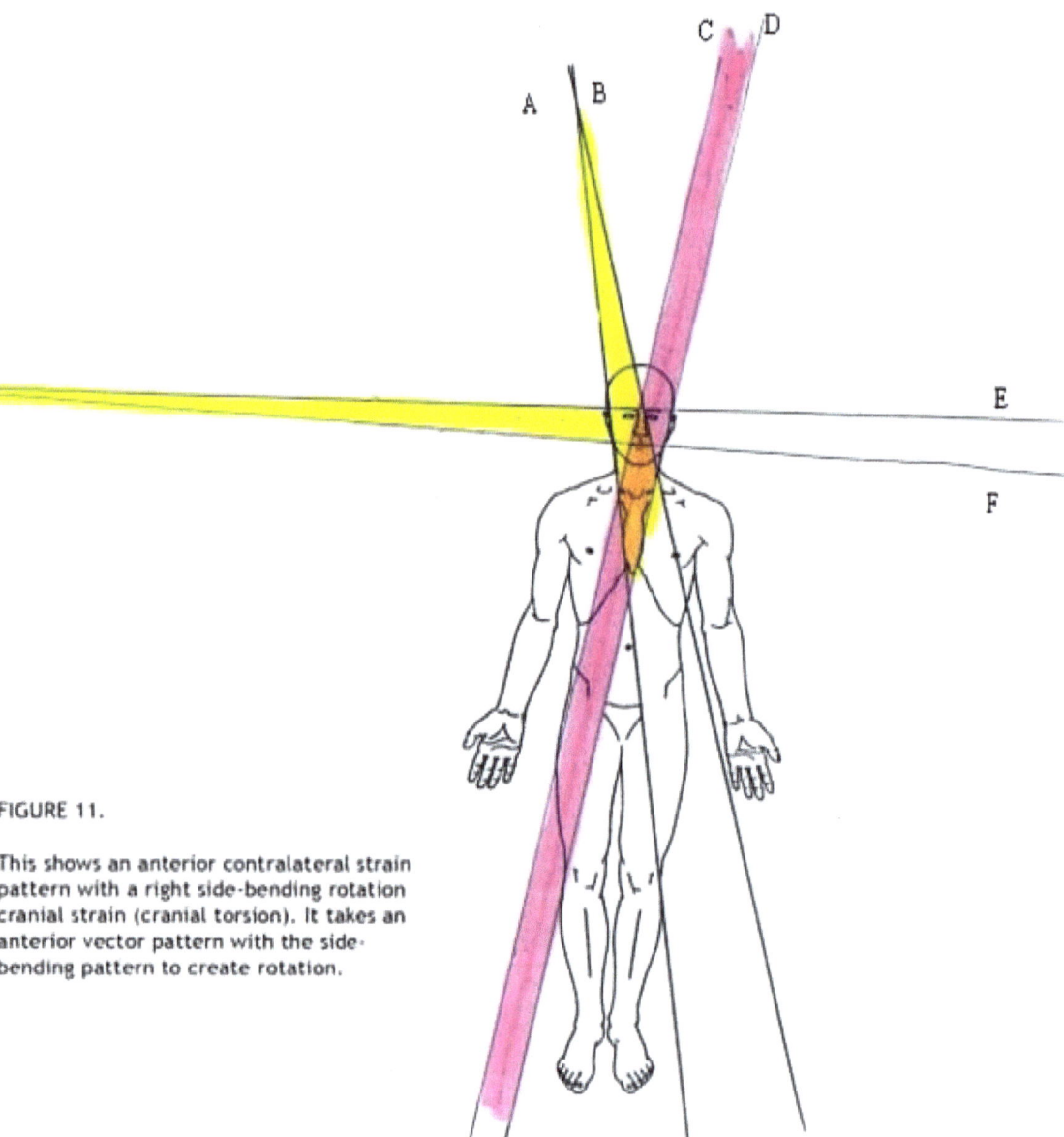

FIGURE 11.

This shows an anterior contralateral strain pattern with a right side-bending rotation cranial strain (cranial torsion). It takes an anterior vector pattern with the side-bending pattern to create rotation.

15

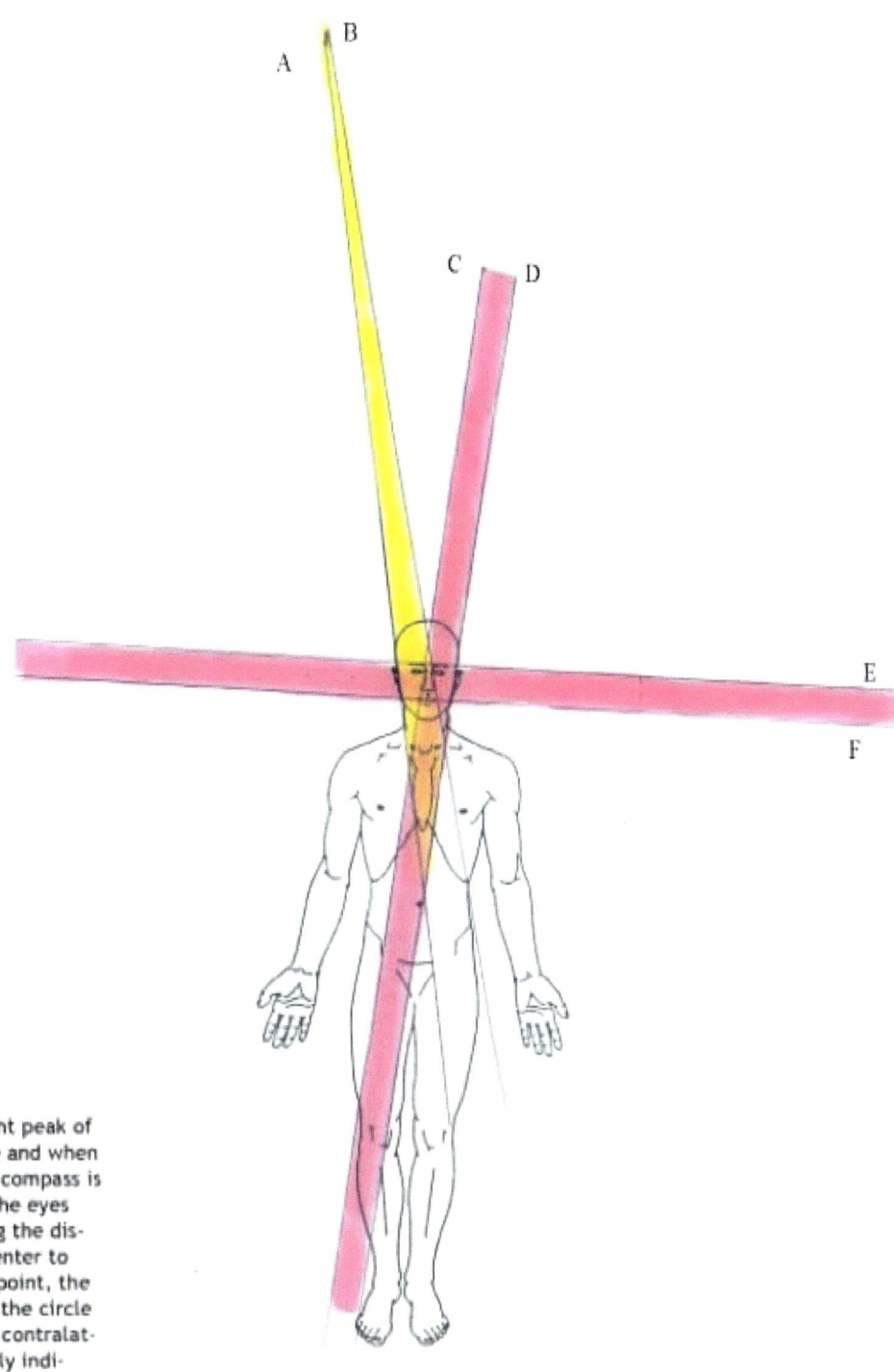

FIGURE 12.

This shows a height peak of the anterior spike and when the center of the compass is placed between the eyes and rotated, using the distance from the center to the convergence point, the circumference of the circle will intersect the contralateral foot. It usually indicates an old navicular problem with subluxation.

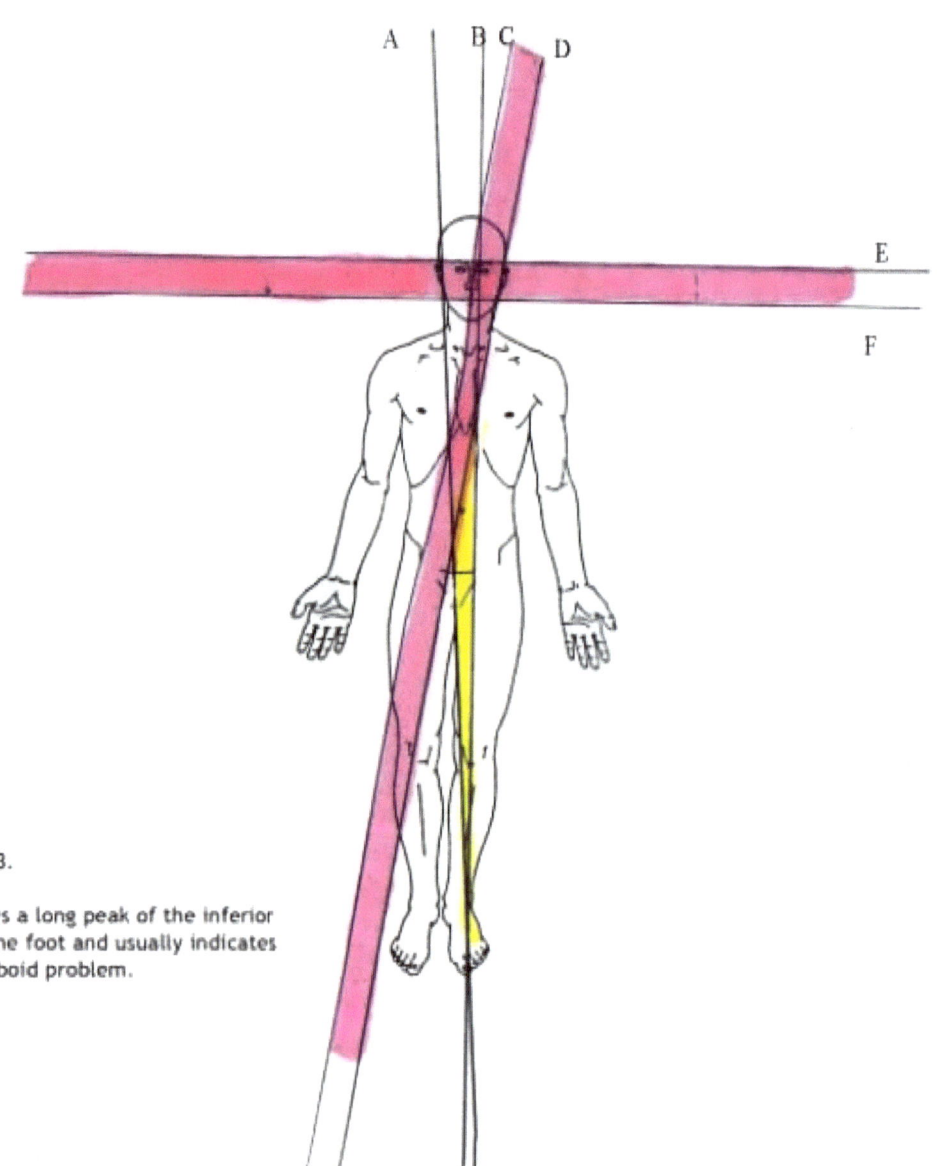

FIGURE 13.

This shows a long peak of the inferior peak at the foot and usually indicates an old cuboid problem.

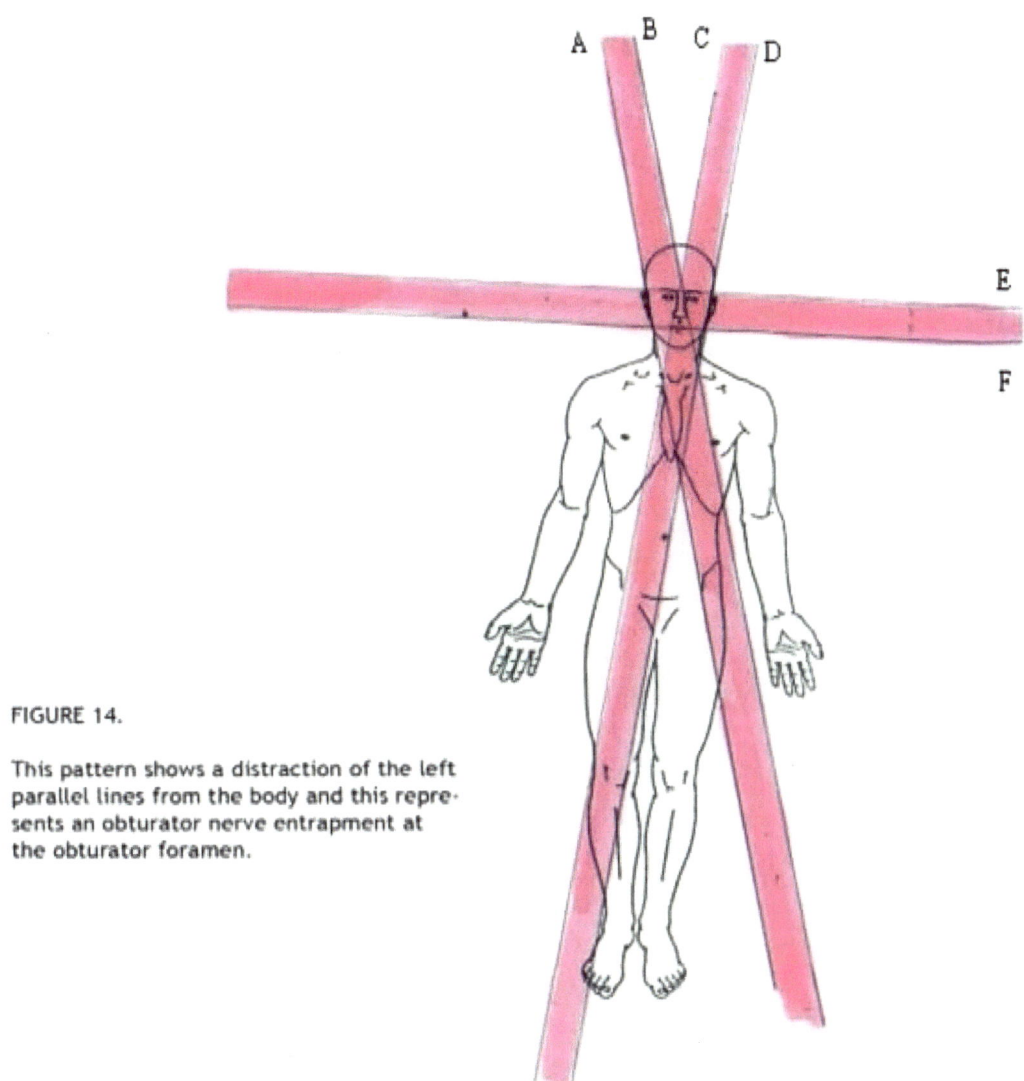

A B C D E F

FIGURE 14.

This pattern shows a distraction of the left parallel lines from the body and this represents an obturator nerve entrapment at the obturator foramen.

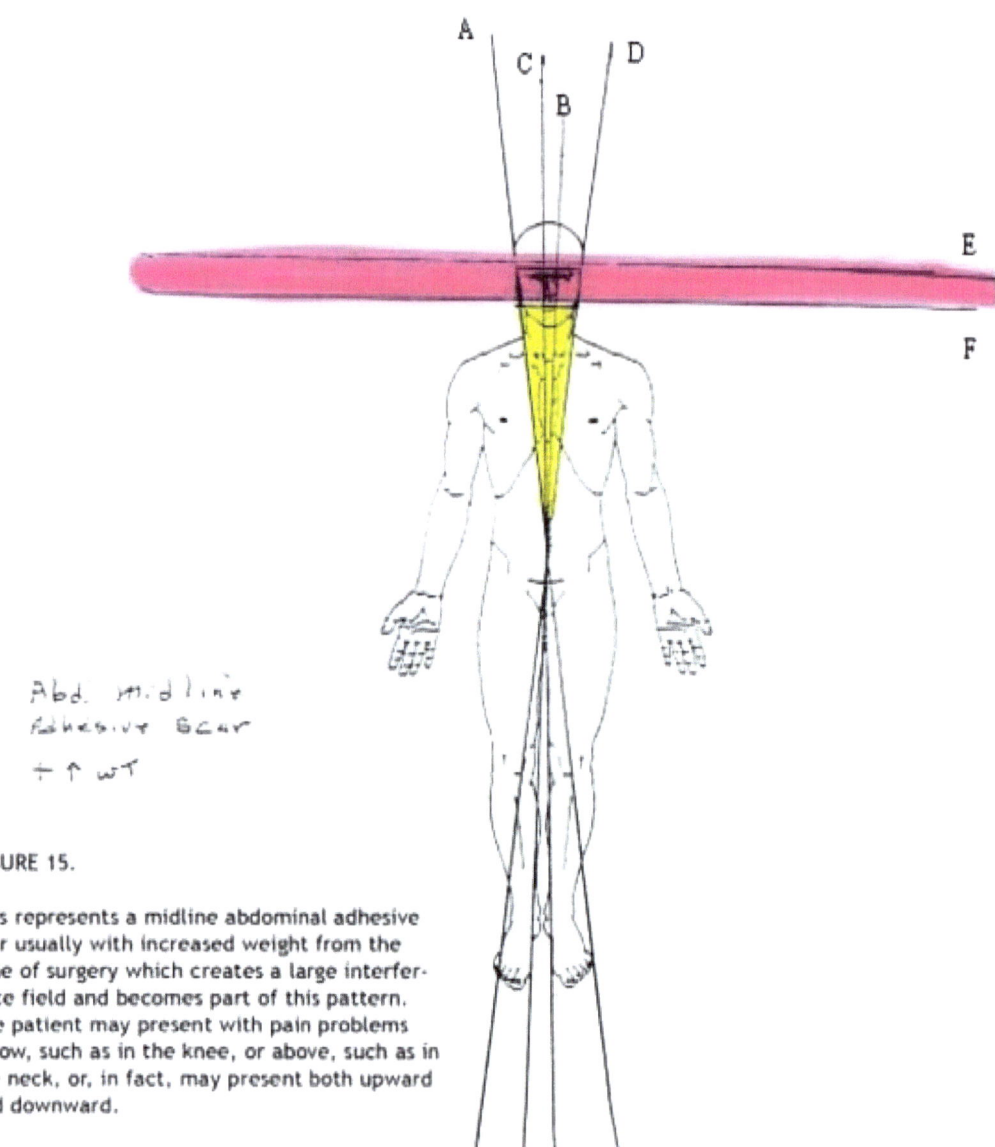

Abd. midline
Adhesive Scar
+ ↑ wt

FIGURE 15.

This represents a midline abdominal adhesive scar usually with increased weight from the time of surgery which creates a large interference field and becomes part of this pattern. The patient may present with pain problems below, such as in the knee, or above, such as in the neck, or, in fact, may present both upward and downward.

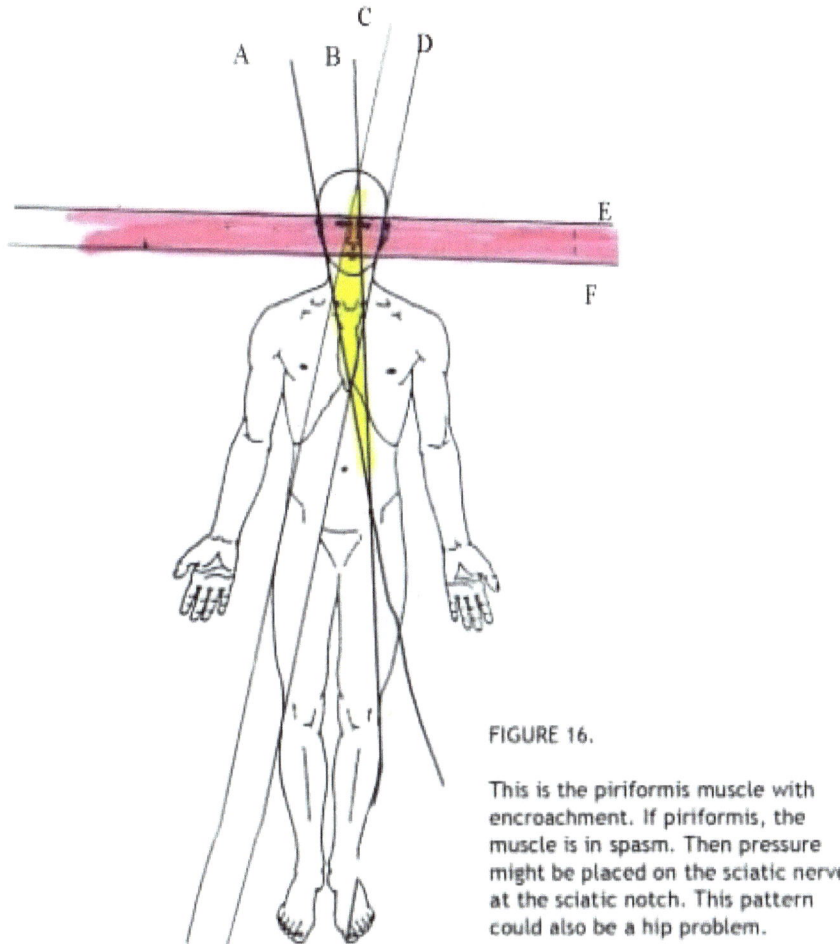

A B C D E F

FIGURE 16.

This is the piriformis muscle with encroachment. If piriformis, the muscle is in spasm. Then pressure might be placed on the sciatic nerve at the sciatic notch. This pattern could also be a hip problem.

Piriformis

20

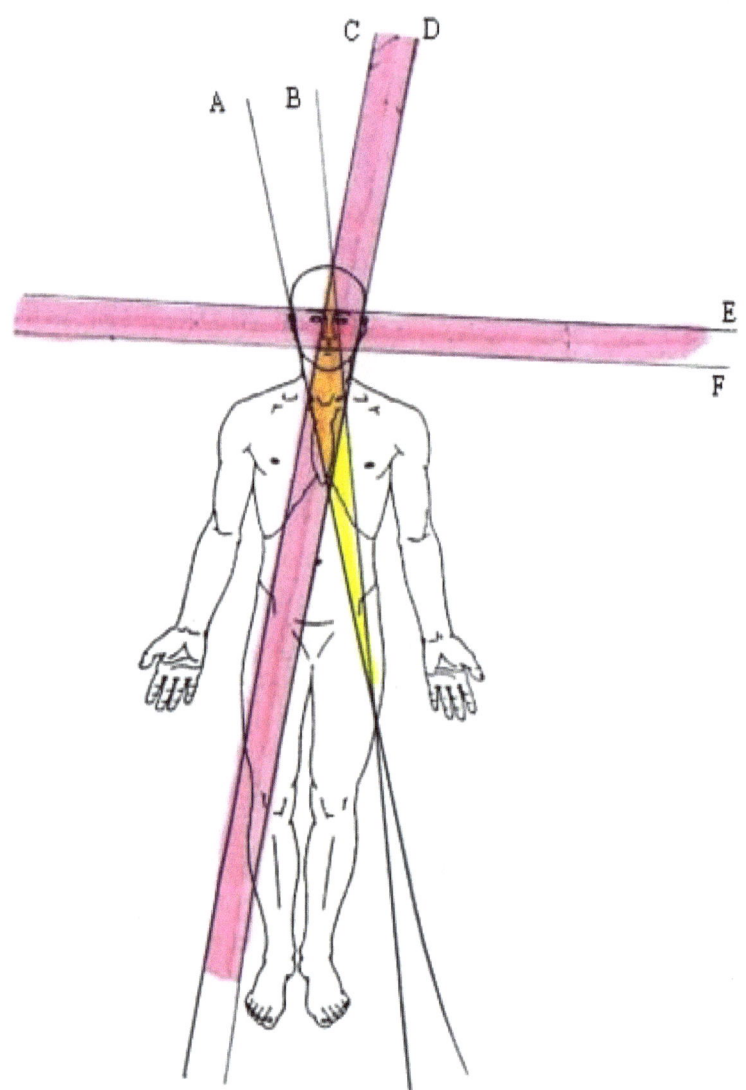

Supra Trochantic Bursitis

FIGURE 17.

This depicts supratrochanteric bursitis with its involvement of the IT (intratrochanteric) band.

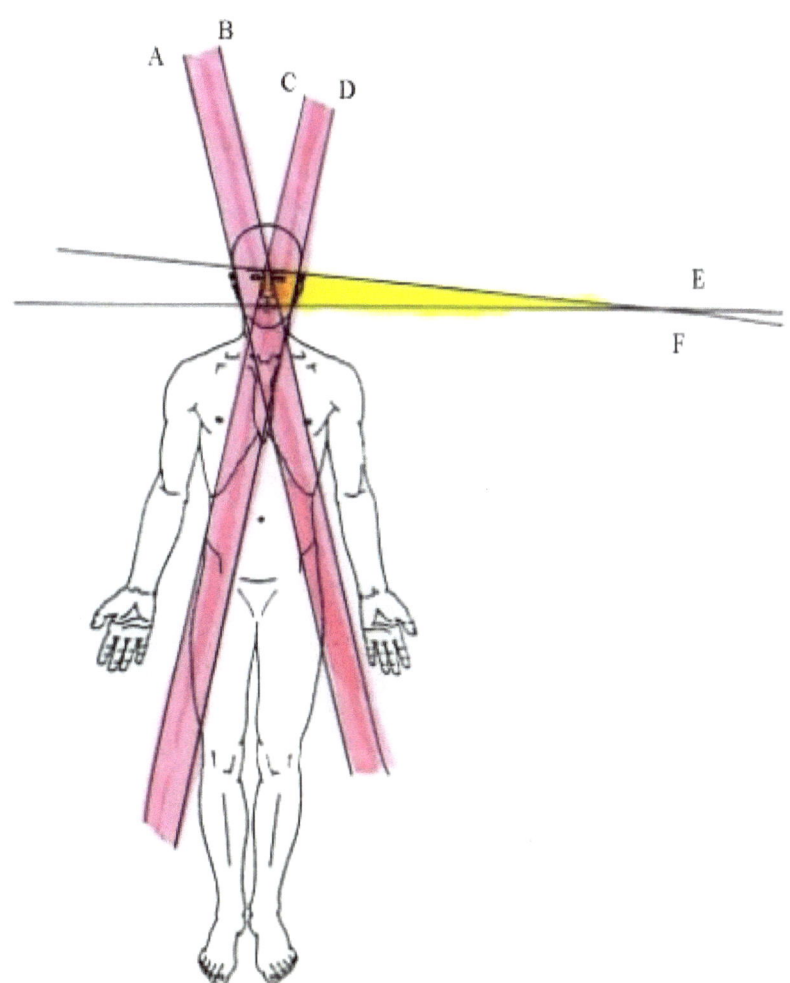

FIGURE 18.

This is a left side-bending cranial strain or dysfunction

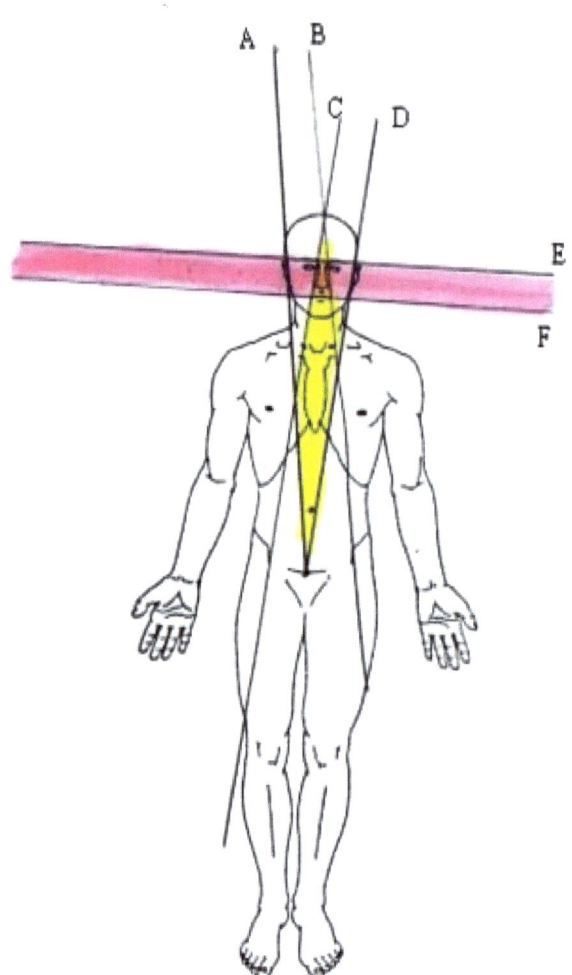

FIGURE 19.

This depicts a pubic symphysis dysfunction. Unlike Figure 5, this pattern is more obvious.

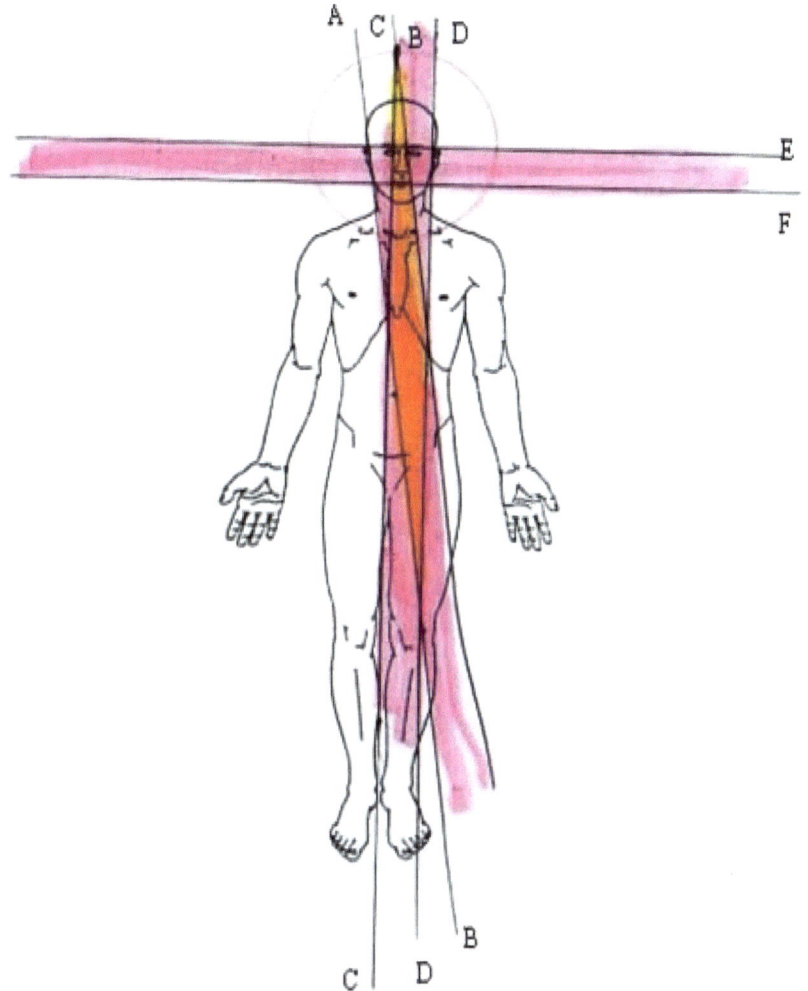

FIGURE 20

This depicts two things. It would depict a knee problem, posterior, from the sciatic side, and would probably involve the hamstring. If we see a convergence above the head, and strike an arc around this patient, we would note a patella or quadricep. Exception to the inferior convergence rule is when lines A & D converge inferiorly which denotes an anterior problem.

24

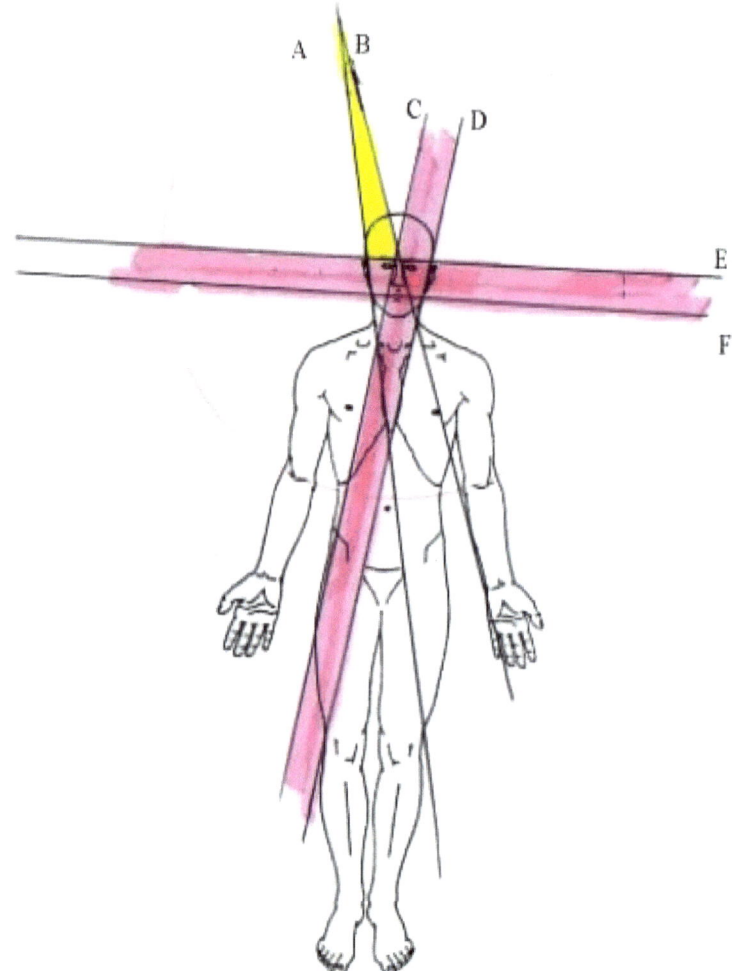

FIGURE 21.

This shows an anterior problem. We can place our compass center between the eyes and strike an arc from the convergent point. This person would probably have an L1 involvement on the left.

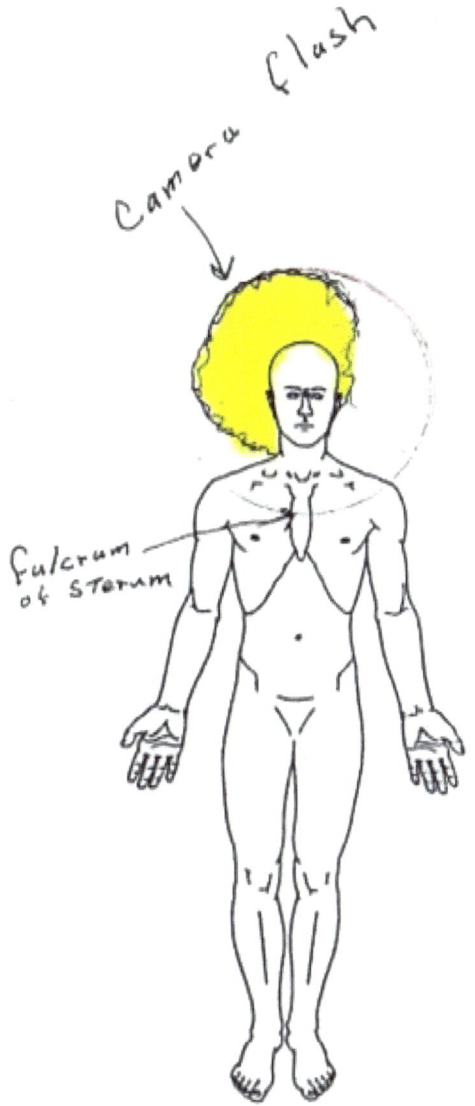

FIGURE 22.

Often when using a Polaroid camera, with a dark background behind the patient, a "flash" or "halo" on the wall will be noted on the photograph around the patient's head. This diagram shows a flash stemming from approximately the fulcrum of the sternum, which is the Angle of Louie, around the skull. When this image appears on the left, usually an abnormaility of some kind can be discovered.

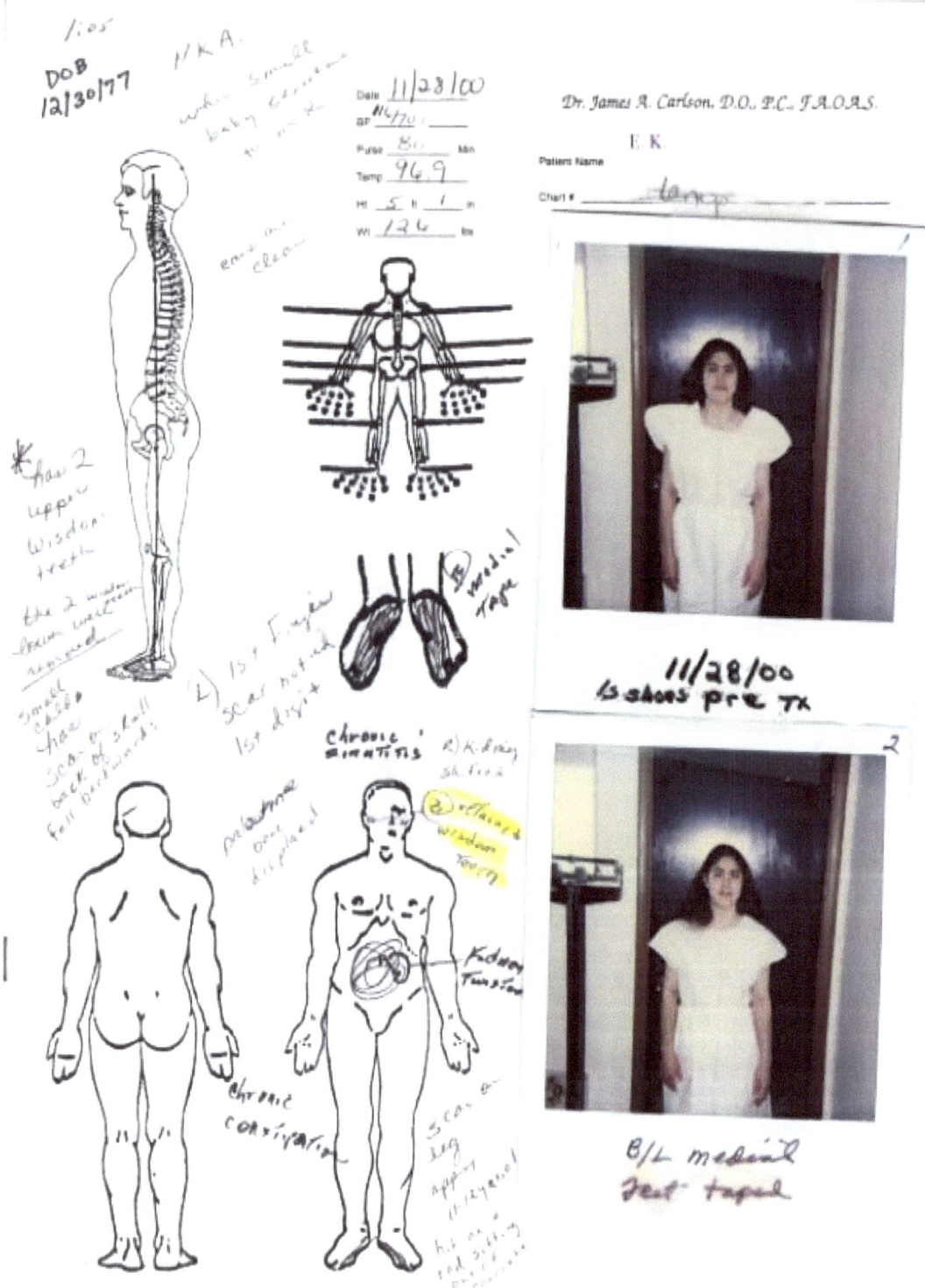

1:05

DOB
12/30/77

N.K.A.

Date 11/28/00
BP 114/70
Purse 80 Min
Temp 96.9
Ht 5 ft 1 in
Wt 126 lbs

Dr. James A. Carlson, D.O., P.C., F.A.O.A.S.

E. K.

Patient Name

Chart # _____

11/28/00
Is shoes pre TX

B/L medial
feet taped

*has 2 upper wisdom teeth

Chronic sinusitis

Kidney
Tumors

Chronic constipation

Dr. James A. Carlson D.O., F.A.O.A.S.

Knoxville, Tennessee 37923
Musculo - Skeletal & Athletic Medicine

E.K.

Patient	11/28/00	Chart #	temp	Page

Date	Progress		Plans

Subj.............................

Has trouble sitting up straight

Slipped & fell on concrete approx 2 yrs ago. - ice Phys and emotional prob, problem c pelvis being tipped forward.

XXX.............................
also Trouble c constipation
Suggested seeing a GI phys
if this tx does not resolve problem.

Will notice after txs previously will feel better for a while & being

X-Ray & Thermography.......
able to stand up straighter but then this will decrease

Lab.............................
when sits in chair

Diagnostic Photos..............

Tx.............................

Dx.............................

Future Plans.....................

Status.............................

Plans:
① New Pt. visit
② Reviewed symptoms c pt.
③ B/L medial feet taped
④ OMT complete c CVS/MFR
⑤ Special cranial tech c CVS/MFR

28

E.K.

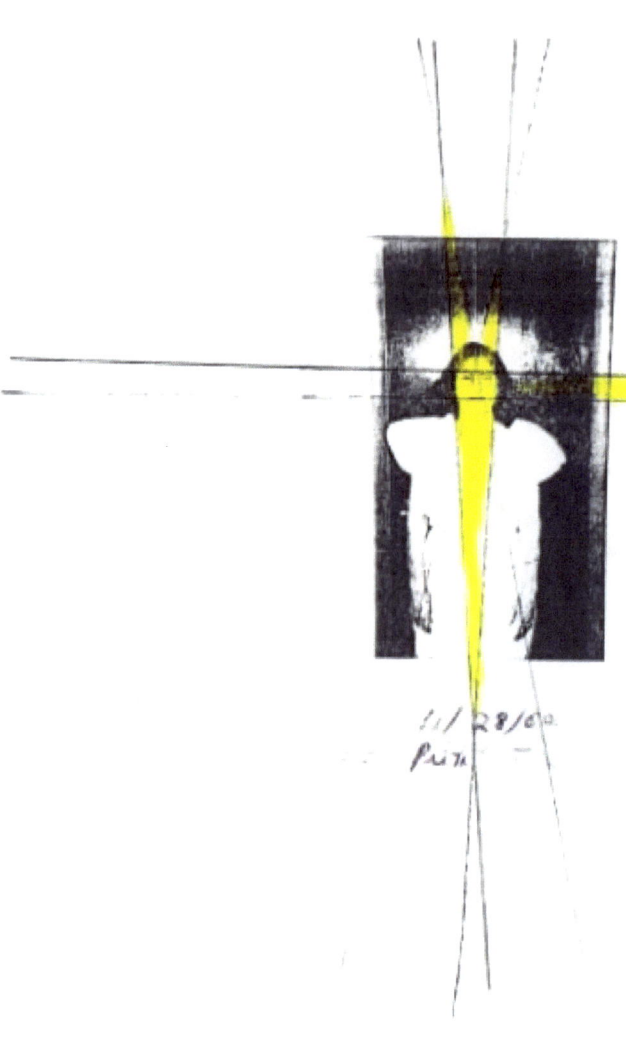

E.K.

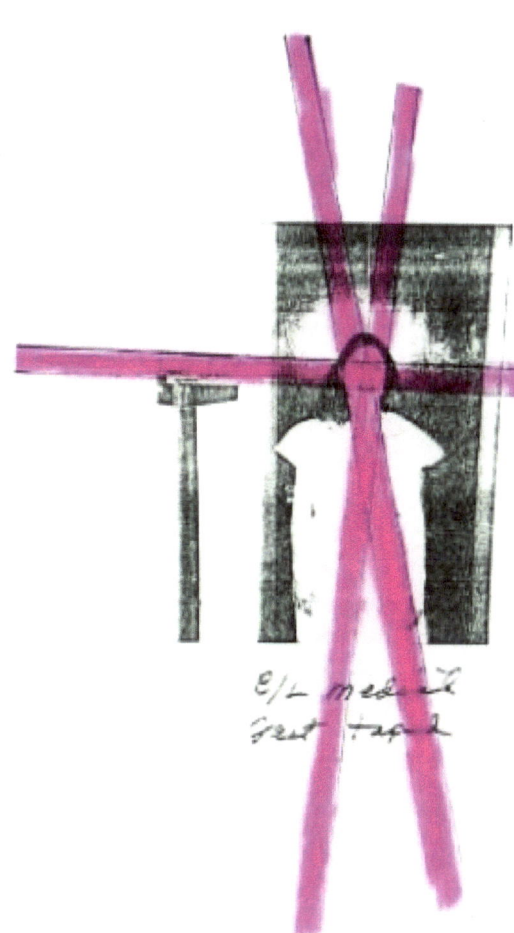

E.K.   11/28/00

This is a 23-year-old Caucasian female who is one of the Amish community. She works in the bakery. Her chief complaint is chronic constipation for the last couple of years. She notes from time to time she does have some burning when she urinates but this is usually around the time of her menstrual period. She tells me during the course of the visit that she has had her two lower wisdom teeth removed but the two uppers are retained and are really compacted. She had several falls and hit the back of her head. She has some scars on her fingers basically and one on her head as well.

Photographs were taken and analyzed and show that she has anterior strain patterns. I did tape and strap her medial feet and this corrected the photographic strain and the patient notes that her balance felt better. I note that her back was slightly discolored from using a heating pad. Her gut was immobile and she had a left kidney that was rotated. She had some sacroiliac dysfunction. She also had some cervical somatic dysfunction and she had a right palatine subluxation. Her craniosacral motion was not there. Her ears were clear. She has been using the candle on her ear to keep them cleaned out. She does teach school. She teaches the fourth grade, six or seven kids, and is a very pleasant young lady. She resides in Ohio and is here on a work program. She complains of chronic sinusitis. She has rather marked dysfunction of the feet.

Treatment today was taping the medial portion of her feet to correct some of the strain while mobilizing the total body, craniosacral, skeletal, extremities, spine and visceral. I have suggested that the patient get her upper wisdom teeth out. I feel this will help not only her chronic sinusitis but well may be the etiology of her constipation. She did mobilize well. She tolerated the procedure well and had some relief following the treatment. I have asked her to return on a p.r.n. basis. JAC:pb

31

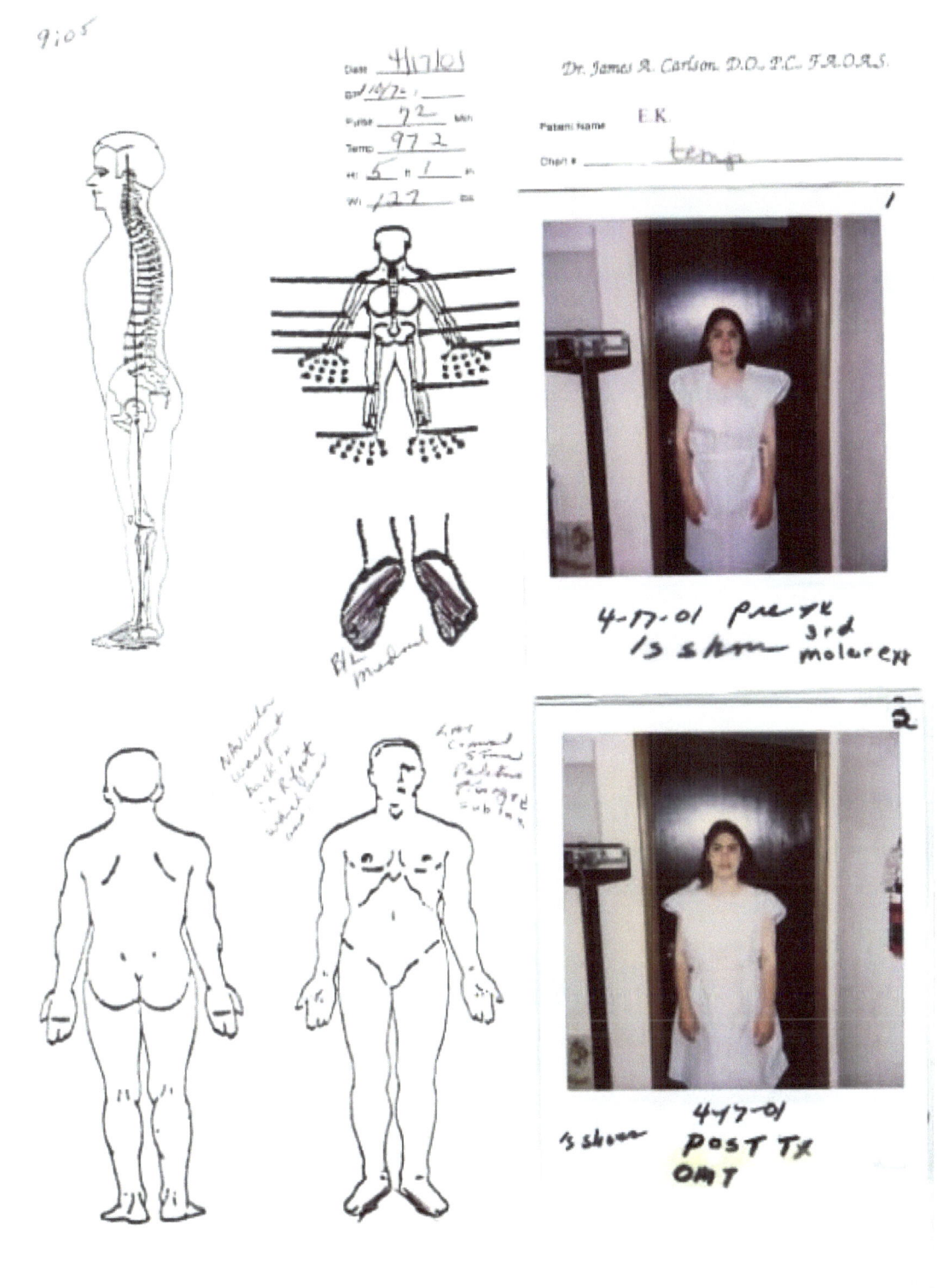

9:05

Date 4/17/01
BP 140/72
Pulse 72 Min
Temp 97 2
Ht 5 ft 1 in
Wt 122 lbs

Dr. James R. Carlson D.O. P.C. F.A.O.A.S.

Patient Name E.K.

Chart # temp

4-17-01 pre tx
is shown 3rd
molar ext

4-17-01
is shown POST TX
OMT

Dr. James A. Carlson D.O., F.A.O.A.S.

Musculo · Skeletal & Athletic Medicine

Patient ___ E.K.   Chart # _tenp_   Page ___

Date _4/17/01_   Progress   Plans

Subj........................

Pt had last 2 upper 3rd
molar removed.
March 16th removal
Notices bite seems to be off
some since dental visit.

XXX........................

X-Ray & Thermography......

Lab........................

Diagnostic Photos..............

Tx........................

Dx........................

Future Plans........................
Status........................

Plans:
1. OMT Comp & Cos/mer
2. Special Cranial
   tech & Cos/mer
3. Diag Photo x2
4. B/L medial fed taped
5.

33

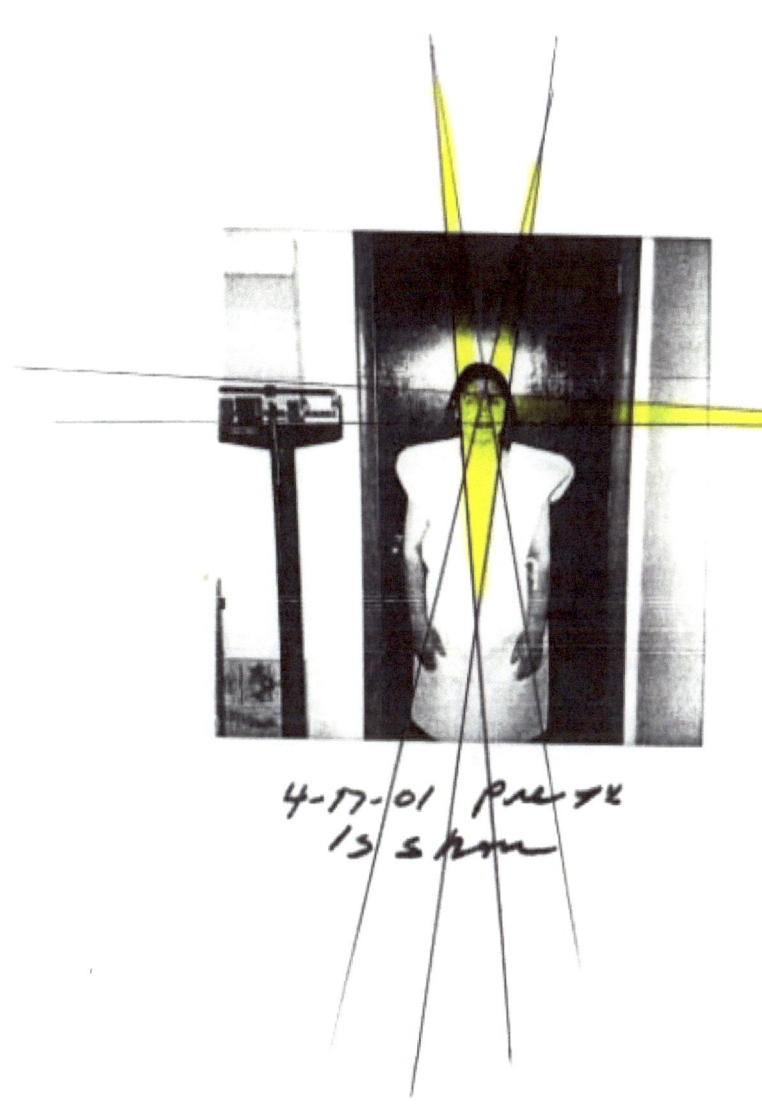

4-17-01 PNE TX
13 5

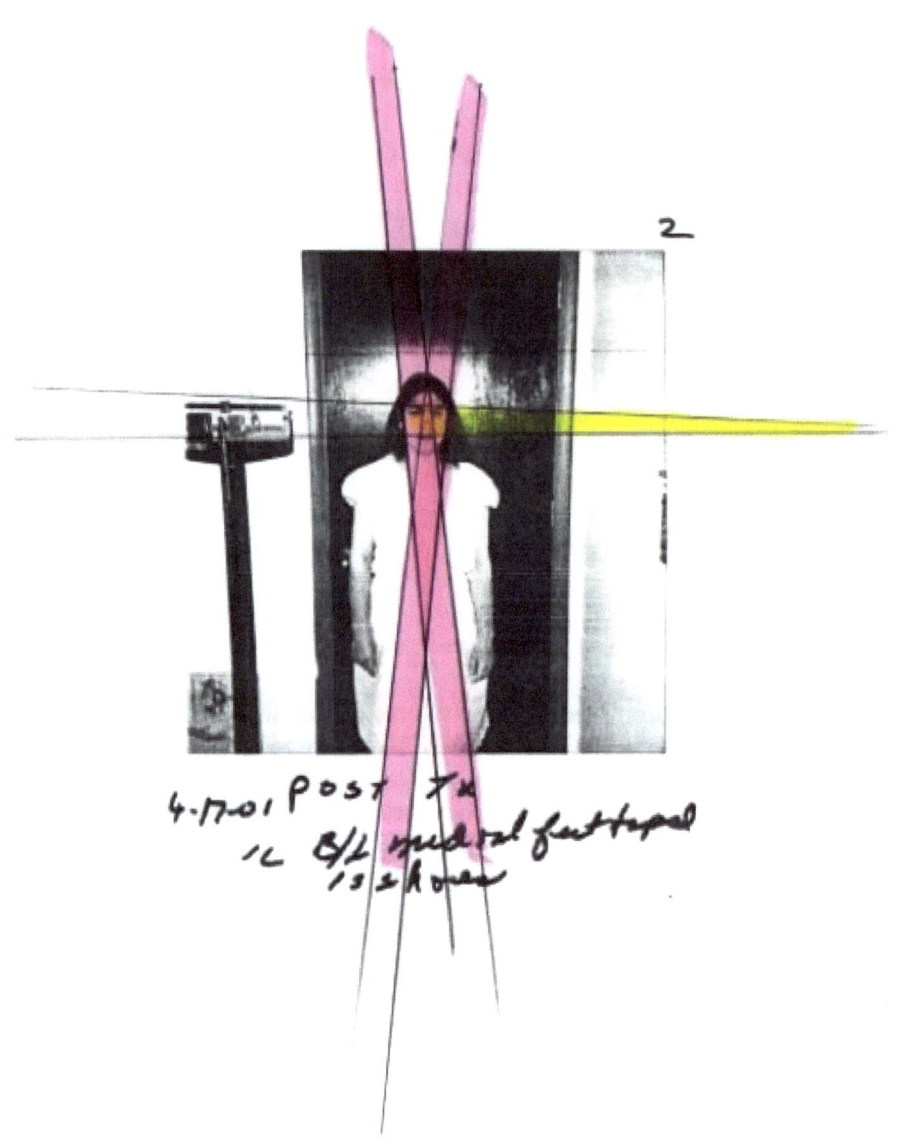

E.K.

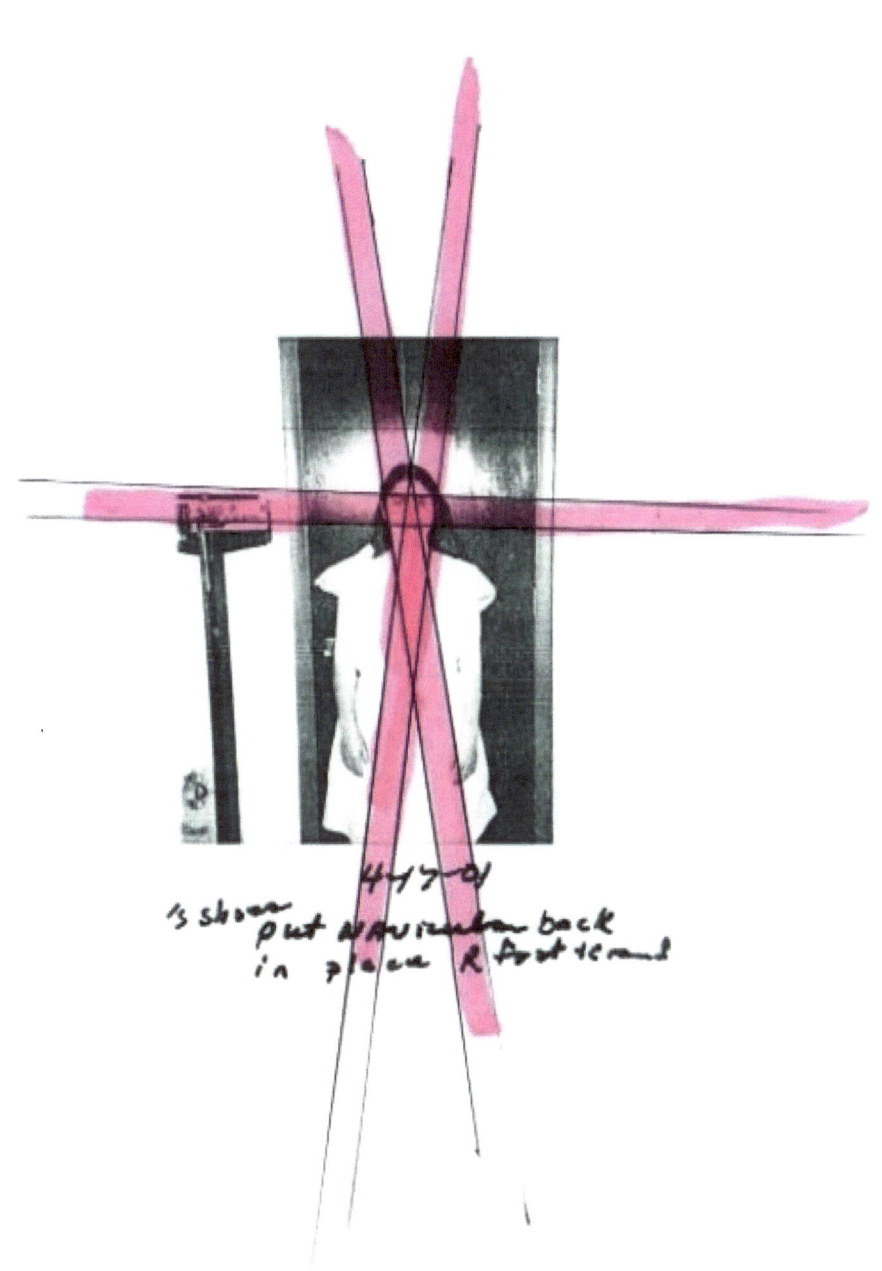

E.K.   04/17/01

She returns today and has had the upper wisdom teeth removed as I had asked. Since she had already had the lower ones out this was creating a strain pattern that could not work through. This strain is shown rather dramatically in the diagnostic photograph. Total mobilization was done to all extremities, the viscera. The side bending rotation of the cranium was treated in a long session. I then repeated the photograph and the long strain patterns were resolved but the lateral strain pattern of the cranium was still present. I taped her feet and she walked around for a while. I went back and redid some of the mobilization of the feet and viscera and finally came back and was able to reduce the cranial strain. Her final photograph would show that this had been accomplished. She had felt some jaw restriction and also some clicking which is consistent with this pattern. She has had constipation and she still has constipation. I feel that some of the visceral cranial strain has caused some of this and this should be better. In general, she appears to be in good health and her attitude is good. She quit her teaching job and is working only in a bakery at this time and this seems to fit her much better.   JAC:pb

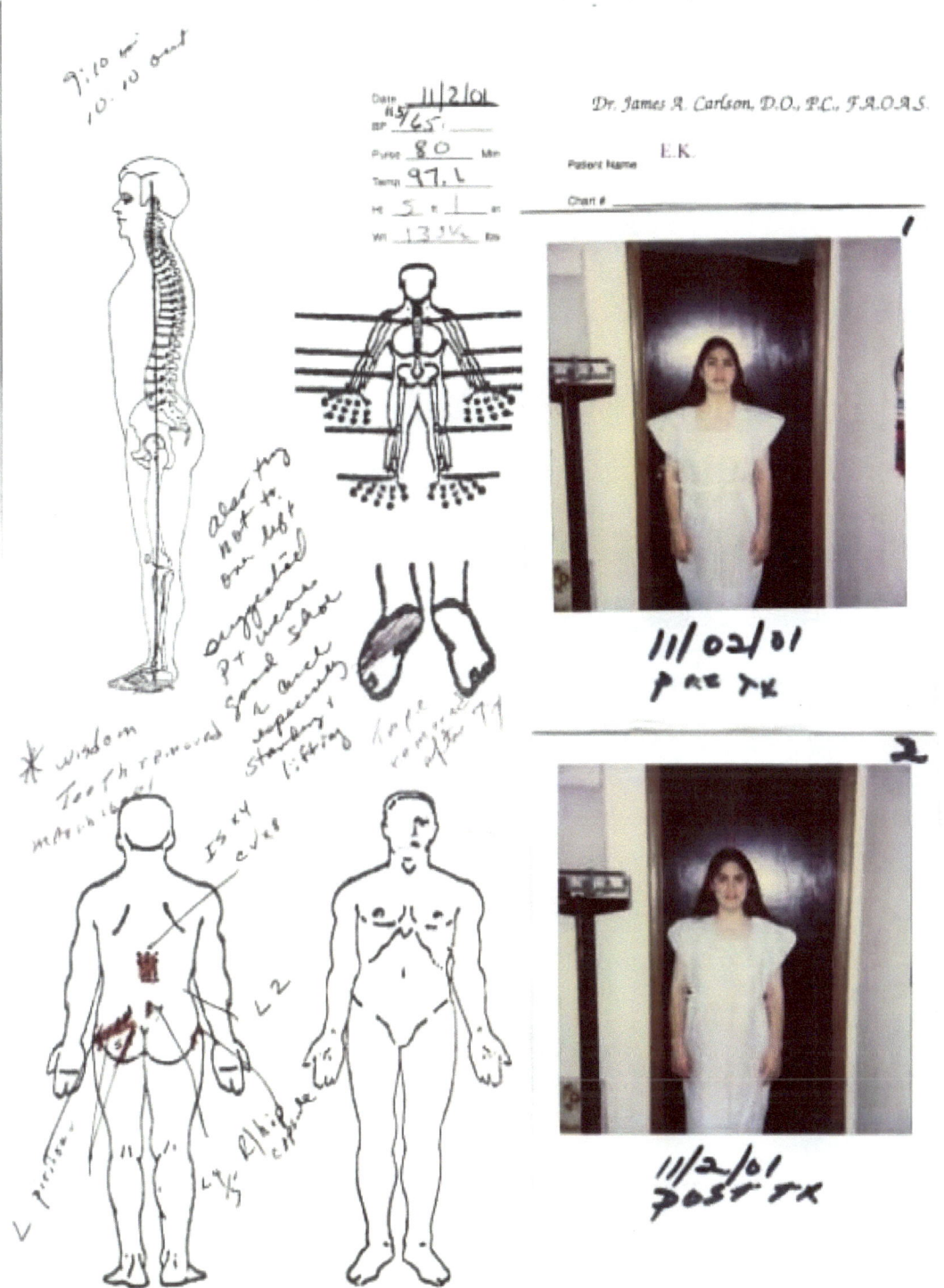

38

Dr. James A. Carlson D.O., F.A.O.A.S.

Musculo - Skeletal & Athletic Medicine

Patient E.K.   Chart # _____   age _____

Date 1/2/01   Progress   Plans

Subj.....................

mid to upper back pain
just recently had a filling placed
which is a composite in the
upper left

① omT Comp & Cas/mfe
② special cranial
    teeth & Cas/mfe
③ Diag Photo
④

XXX...........................

X-Ray & Thermography......

Lab................................

Diagnostic Photos.............

Tx..................................

Dx..................................

Future Plans.....................

Status.............................

E.K.

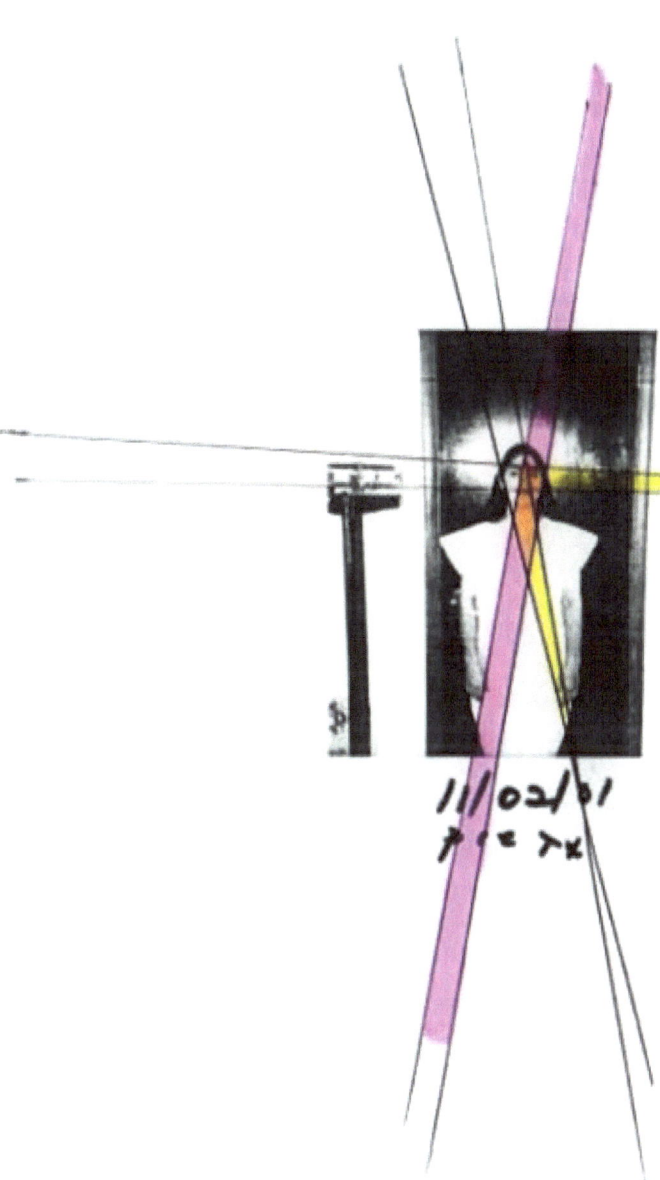

11/02/01
Pre TX

40

E.K.

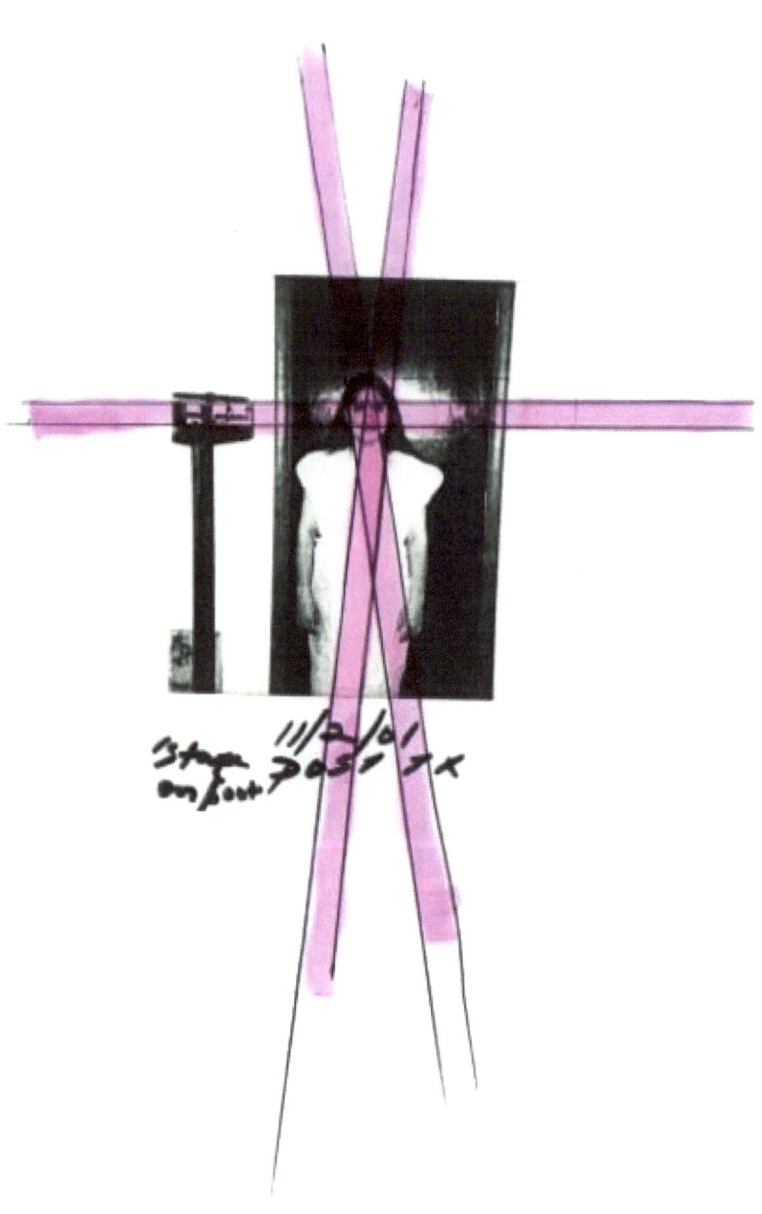

10:00 am

Date 10/16/02

BP 11965

Pulse 80 min

Temp 958

Ht 5 7

Wt 116½

Dr. James A. Carlson, D.O., P.C., F.A.O.A.S.

Patient Name E S

Chart # 8935

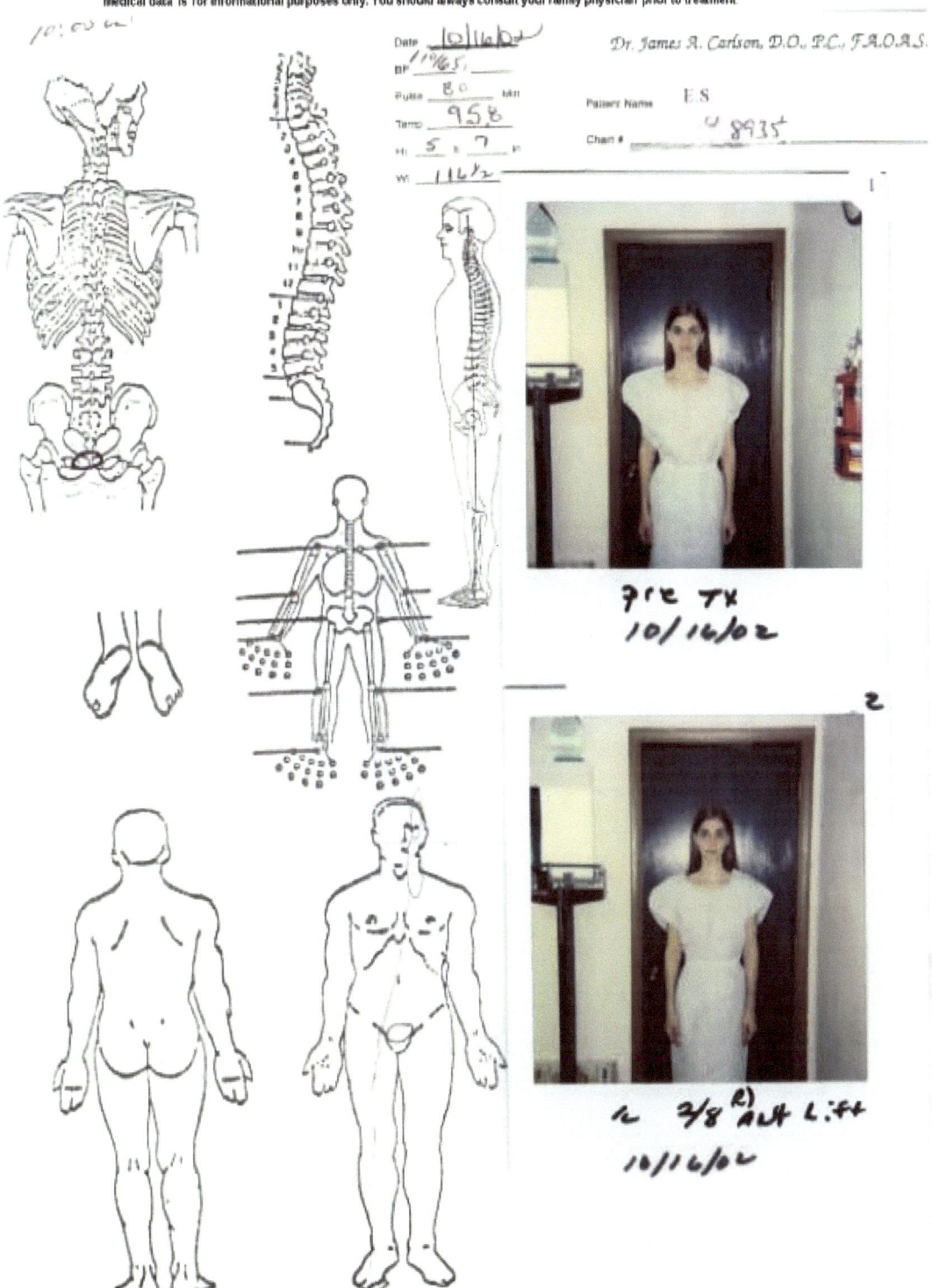

Pre TX
10/16/02

¾ (R) Alt Lift
10/16/02

42

James A. Carlson D.O.P.C.
800 N. CEDAR BLUFF ROAD
KNOXVILLE, TENNESSEE 37923
Musculo-Skeletal & Athletic Medicine

PATIENT E.S.	CHART # 8935	PAGE
DATE 10/16/02 PROGRESS		PLANS

Pt seen today f/a H/As age 19
H/A's 1st) age 14 felt like someone threw a
brick @ pt. Helping father roof a house
in S. Carolina. Grandparent on Father side have
adult onset Diabetes.
Dizzi~~ started @ 9 yrs old
Father is a retired Marine
Artillery officer.
Always gets dizzy the day before
H/A occur. Starts in neck, more of an ache + throb
enters left side of head. Chews only on the left side
Forceps baby
Pt does not have a H/A at this time as they usually start at 3:00 PM;
legs cramping spring, summer Charly horse
in Q leg.
notices cracking in jaw
When sun rises headache resolves usually around 5 PM
Massage helps @ the time only

Pt is a UT student, architecture

Dancing fell several years ago + hit on back.
Spurring noticed on X-Ray

PLANS

① New Pt history
② OMT Compr.
C & S / MFR
③ Special cranial
tx & S & S/MFR
④ Review X-Rays
in pt taken 8/10/02
⑤ Lifts placed
on the R/AW ⅞ X2
⑥ Pt given a
copy of public
Symphysis

Pt wanted to wait
+ call her mother
who lives in Maryland
she was not @ home
called from the tx
room

E.S.

Pt Now had ↑↑ S. listed

① Message

② Saw an Osteopath in Washington D.C.
Scott ~~Kawasaki~~ appro 4 visits. This did help
Kwiat Kowski DO
last appr 2 wks ~~~~ did & this wean out

Pt is

44

Dr. James A. Carlson, D.O., P.C., F.A.O.A.S.

509 N. Cedar Bluff Rd. • Knoxville, Tennessee 37923

Name E.S.   Patient 8935   Date 10/16/02

Scar (approximate weight at time of scar) _____ lbs. _____ date

Billfold: ❑ (Right) none or ❑ (Left) Hip	Bra ✔ Hat ❑ rarely	Belt ❑ rarely
Hair Piece ❑ none Hair up tight ❑ only when dancing	Rings: ❑ (Right) occasional or ❑ (Left)	or ❑ (Both)
Shoe Lifts ❑ none High Heels ❑	Dentures ❑ Braces ❑	Bridges ❑
Wrist Watch: ❑ (Right) or ❑ (Left) handed	Glasses: ❑ Full Time ❑ Part Time Last Eye Exam _____	

Pt is right handed
45 years age
NO surgeries
Pt does have a lot of crowns
Crowns + 1 drilling + filling appt 4 dental fillings

glasses driving only
dental braces
1 age 10
2nd set 15 age
age 16 jaw locked
for 11 days
jaw unlocked the following day
braces removed

NO wisdom teeth

pt has had t&s listed
(1) massage
(2) saw osteopath in Washington, D.C.
(3) Dr. _____, about 4 visits, which helped.
(5) more out in about 2 weeks

What are your expectations of your visit with Dr. Carlson today? _____

45

HEALTHSOUTH
Diagnostic Center of Knoxville
601 Hall of Fame Dr.
Knoxville, TN 37915

865-525-7100 Business Office
865-525-7000 Scheduling
865-525-7797 Medical Records

Account #: 141198   Our Courier

Name: E.S.

Home Phone: Deleted
Work Phone:

Date of Birth: 7/28/83 Sex: F

Ref: 01678 JAMES CARLSON

Date of Procedure: 10/10/02

STANDING PELVIC RADIOGRAPHS:

Two views of the pelvis were obtained in the standing position. There are
no bony or soft tissue abnormalities. Specifically, there are no fractures
or osseous lesions.

IMPRESSION:

1. Negative study.

                    GLENN E.   JUNG, M.D./nr

46

Medical data is for informational purposes only. You should always consult your family physician prior to treatment.

appt. 10-16-02 Wed.
10:00
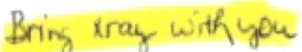
Bring xray with you

PATIENT REGISTRATION FORM
James A. Carlson, D.O., P.C., F.A.O.A.S.
947-0548

PATIENT INFORMATION *(Please write information about the patient here.)*   **DATE:**

PATIENT'S NAME (Last, First Middle Initial)	SEX	REFERRING DOCTOR
E.S.	☐ Male ☒ Female	Dr. Scott Kwiatkowski

PATIENT'S ADDRESS	REFERRING DOCTOR ADDRESS	CITY	STATE	ZIP
Deleted	suite #4	Bethesda	MD	

CITY	STATE	ZIP	EMPLOYER'S NAME	TELEPHONE
Deleted				( )

TELEPHONE	MARITAL STATUS	DATE OF BIRTH	EMPLOYER'S ADDRESS	CITY	STATE	ZIP
865	☒ Single ☐ Married · ☐ Separated ☐ Divorce ☐ Widowed	2/8/83 MO DAY YR				

AGE	SOCIAL SECURITY NUMBER	DRIVERS LICENSE NUMBER	EMPLOYMENT STATUS	STUDENT STATUS: If 19 Years or Older:
19			☐ Full Time ☐ Retired ☐ Part Time ☒ Not Employed	☒ Full Time ☐ Part Time ☐ Not a Student

MEDICARE PATIENTS ONLY

NAME AS IT APPEARS ON YOUR MEDICARE CARD:_____ MEDICARE ID #:_____
Please be sure to give us your Medicare Card so we may make a copy of it to include with your medical records.

AUTHORIZATION TO PAY BENEFITS AND RELEASE OF INFORMATION

I request that payment of authorized Medicare benefits be made either to me or on my behalf to James A. Carlson, D.O., P.C., F.A.O.A.S. for any services furnished me by that physician. I authorize any holder of medical information needed to determine these benefits or the benefits payable for related services.

I request and authorize James A. Carlson, D.O., P.C., F.A.O.A.S. to inquire of Medicare, in my behalf, in regard to their payment of benefits on charges by James A. Carlson, D.O., P.C., F.A.O.A.S.

Signature:_____   Date:_____

FINANCIAL POLICY

PRIVATE INSURANCE OR INSURANCE PROVIDED BY YOUR EMPLOYER: We do not participate with any of the Managed Care programs, nor do we accept assignment from any insurance carrier. *ALL PATIENTS ARE TO PAY FOR SERVICES AT TIME OF VISIT, REGARDLESS OF INSURANCE COVERAGE.*

MEDICARE: We do not accept Medicare assignments, however, we are required by federal law to file Medicare claims on your behalf. Medicare benefits will be paid directly to you. Therefore, we ask that all patients pay for their visits at time of service.

MEDICAID/TENNCARE: We are not a Medicaid/Tenncare provider. Therefore, if you are insured by Medicaid/Tenncare we will not be able to treat you, nor will we be able to treat you as a private/personal pay patient, as this is a violation of Tennessee law.

RETURNED CHECKS: If your bank returns your check to us unpaid, a $15.00 penalty will be assessed to you.

ALL PATIENTS PLEASE READ AND SIGN: I have read the above FINANCIAL POLICY, understand it, and agree to comply with its terms. If litigation, on other collection means are used to collect any unpaid balance, I agree to pay all attorney fees and/or other costs of collecting.

Signature:_____   Date: 9/25/02

HOW DID YOU HEAR ABOUT US?	Through Dr. Scott Kwiatkowski P.O., P.C. practicing in Bethesda MD

IN CASE OF AN EMERGENCY - WHO SHOULD WE CONTACT? - (Please list someone living at a residence other than those listed on the reverse side)	NAME: Deleted ADDRESS: ___ CITY: ___ STATE: ___	TELEPHONE: DAY Deleted cell night RELATIONSHIP Mother

47

PATIENT HEALTH HISTORY

Name _____   Sex **F**   Age **19**

Referred by ___ **E.S.** _____

PLEASE CHECK ALL PAST OR PRESENT SYMPTOMS WHICH APPLY TO YOU. *(If you don't recognize the term, you probably haven't had it.)*

Past Present Category

HEART PROBLEMS
- ☐ ☐ heart attack
- ☒ ☐ heart or chest pain
- ☐ ☐ tachycardia (heartbeat racing)
- ☐ ☐ abnormal EKG (Electrocardiogram)
- ☐ ☐ heart murmur
- ☐ ☐ partial heart block
- ☐ ☐ endocarditis
- ☐ ☐ angina
- ☐ ☐ high blood pressure
- ☐ ☐ low blood pressure

SKIN PROBLEMS
- ☐ ☐ unexplained rashes
- ☐ ☐ excessive itching
- ☐ ☐ red flushes of color
- ☐ ☐ rough skin
- ☒ ☒ acne (pimples)

NERVOUS DISORDERS
- ☐ ☐ Multiple Sclerosis
- ☐ ☐ Bell's palsy
- ☐ ☐ shingles (herpes zoster)
- ☐ ☐ numbness in any part of body
- ☐ ☐ tingling in any part of body
- ☐ ☐ epilepsy or convulsions
- ☐ ☐ Dr. told you "it's your nerves"
- ☐ ☐ the shakes of hands, feet, head, etc.
- ☐ ☐ twitching of face or other muscles
- ☐ ☐ knee or leg jerks, especially at night

DIGESTION
(Gastrointestinal Disorders)
- ☐ ☐ diverticulitis
- ☐ ☐ ulcers
- ☐ ☐ Crohn's disease
- ☐ ☐ Graves' disease
- ☐ ☐ indigestion
- ☐ ☐ bloated feeling after eating
- ☐ ☐ heartburn
- ☐ ☐ poor appetite
- ☐ ☐ diarrhea
- ☐ ☐ constipation

BLOOD DISEASES
- ☐ ☐ mononucleosis
- ☐ ☐ false positive for venereal disease

CANCER
- ☐ ☐ leukemia
- ☐ ☐ Hodgkin's disease
- ☐ ☐ any other (name) _____

ENDOCRINE PROBLEMS
- ☐ ☐ thyroid — underactive or overactive
- ☐ ☐ pancreas
- ☐ ☐ diabetes
- ☐ ☐ ovaries
- ☐ ☐ testes
- ☐ ☐ menstruation — painful, too often or too seldom, stopping without reason
- ☐ ☐ hysterectomy — complete
- ☐ ☐ tipped uterus
- ☐ ☐ cervical erosion
- ☐ ☐ prostate problem
- ☐ ☐ overweight
- ☐ ☐ underweight
- ☐ ☐ chronically subnormal temperature

EMOTIONAL
- ☐ ☐ sudden anger
- ☐ ☐ depression
- ☐ ☐ wish you were dead
- ☐ ☐ irritability
- ☐ ☐ suicidal tendencies
- ☐ ☐ been divorced

ANNOYING SYMPTOMS
- ☐ ☐ metallic taste in mouth
- ☒ ☐ frequent headaches
- ☐ ☐ noises in your ears
- ☐ ☐ ringing in your ears
- ☐ ☐ hissing in your ears
- ☐ ☐ chronic eye inflammation
- ☐ ☐ chronic fatigue
- ☐ ☐ do you tire easily
- ☐ ☐ swollen lymph nodes
- ☐ ☐ hearing problems
- ☐ ☐ do you sweat excessively
- ☐ ☐ cold hands and feet
- ☐ ☐ motion sickness
- ☐ ☐ slow healing
- ☒ ☐ leg cramps
- ☐ ☒ dizziness
- ☐ ☐ get up at night to urinate
- ☐ ☐ urinate frequently during the day
- ☒ ☐ have insomnia
- ☐ ☐ tired when awaken in morning
- ☐ ☐ have trouble making decisions
- ☐ ☐ burning sensation in mouth
- ☐ ☐ increased flow of saliva
- ☐ ☐ sore throat, no infection present

ALLERGIES
- ☐ ☐ metals — like copper, nickel _____
- ☐ ☐ fabrics _____
- ☐ ☐ soaps & detergents _____
- ☐ ☐ other _____

DISEASES
- ☐ ☐ arthritis; rheumatoid, osteoid
- ☐ ☐ bursitis
- ☐ ☐ tennis elbow
- ☐ ☐ painful joints
- ☐ ☐ Friedreich's ataxia
- ☐ ☐ asthma
- ☐ ☐ surgery (for what) _____
- ☐ ☐ osteomyelitis
- ☐ ☐ psoriasis
- ☐ ☐ sickle cell anemia
- ☐ ☐ chronic anemia
- ☐ ☐ kidney stones

MISCELLANEOUS
- ☐ ☐ infections take long time to heal
- ☐ ☐ do you work around mercury — (what capacity)
- ☐ ☐ what medications are you taking — _____

DENTAL HISTORY
- ☐ ☐ silver amalgam fillings in mouth
- ☐ ☐ gold fillings in mouth
- ☐ ☐ removable metal bridge in mouth
- ☐ ☐ gold bridge in mouth
- ☐ ☐ porcelain/gold crowns in mouth
- ☐ ☐ non-precious crowns in mouth
- ☐ ☐ porcelain / semi or non-precious crowns in mouth
- ☐ ☐ root canal
- ☐ ☐ more than half your teeth removed
- ☐ ☐ periodontal (gum) disease

GENERAL HISTORY
- ☐ ☐ vegetarian
- ☐ ☐ smoke tobacco products
- ☒ ☐ take calcium supplements
- ☐ ☐ take bone meal or dolomite
- ☐ ☐ eat saltwater fish once/week or more
- ☐ ☐ eat shell fish once/week or more
- ☐ ☐ drink coffee
- ☐ ☐ avoid salt
- ☐ ☐ avoid butter and other fats

PATIENT PAIN DRAWING

Name   E.S.   Date 9/25/02

Mark the areas on your body where you feel the sensations decribed below, using the appropriate symbol. Mark the areas of radiation. Include all affected areas.

Aching	Numbness	Pins and needles	Burning	Stabbing
▲▲▲		000	xxx	///

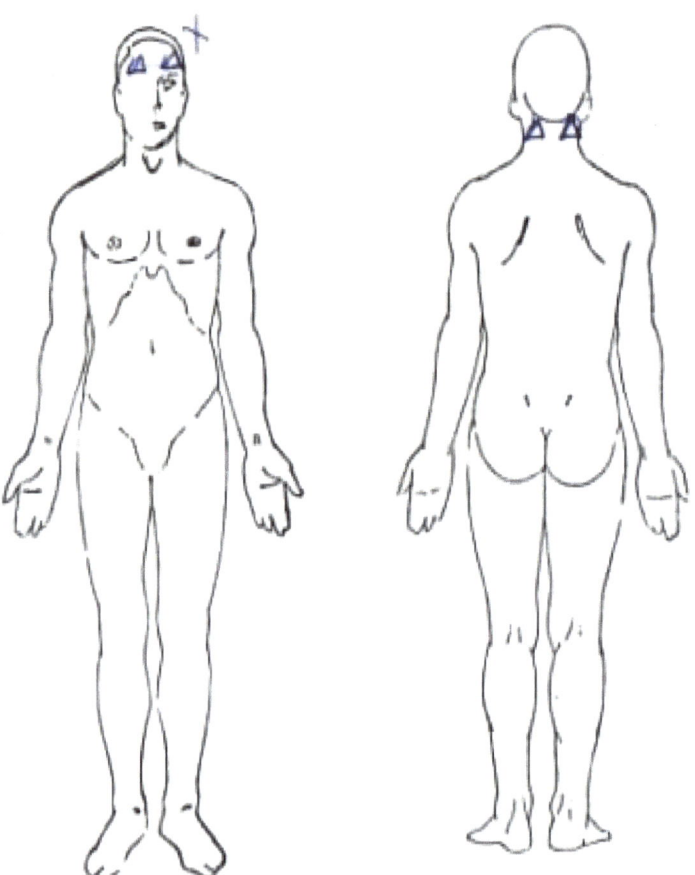

Please mark with an X, on the drawing above, at the location where the pain is worst now.
How bad is your pain now? Please mark on the line below how bad your pain is now.

No pain <-----|-----|-----|-----|-----|-----|-----|-----|-----|-----|-----|-----|-----|-----|-----|----->Worst possible pain

49

PATIENT HISTORY QUESTIONNAIRE

Name: E.S.　　　　　　　　　　　　　Age: 19　　Occupation: Student (Architecture)

PRESENT STATUS

1. When (roughly what date) did your present pain start? _July_
   Are you still working? ❑ yes ❑ no　Last day on job _____

2. A. Where did the pain start? _head_
   B. Where did the pain spread to? _neck_
   C. Does the pain ☒ throb ❑ twinge ❑ burn?
   D. How did pain start? (check appropriate box)
   ☒ suddenly　　　☒ gradually　　　❑ lifting　　　❑ twisting
   ❑ fall　　　❑ bending　　　❑ pulling　　　❑ injured during sports
   ❑ injured in auto accident　❑ hit from behind　☒ no apparent cause

3. What activities make the pain worse?
   ❑ during exercise　❑ after exercise　❑ sitting　❑ standing
   ❑ walking　❑ bending forward　❑ bending backward　❑ coughing
   ❑ sneezing　❑ other _____

4. A. Is the Pain worse in the ❑ AM ☒ PM?
   B. Can you get comfortable at night? ❑ yes ❑ no　(see 5K below) _Depends_
   C. How does your back feel in the morning? ☒ stiff ❑ sore ❑ fine
   D. Once you get started moving about, does it ❑ worsen? ☒ ease?
   E. What is it like at the end of the day? ❑ worse ❑ easier _depends_
   F. What reduces/eases the pain? ❑ lying down ❑ sitting ☒ massage
   ❑ standing ❑ walking ❑ manipulation ❑ exercises in physical therapy
   ❑ pain pills ❑ injection for pain ❑ aspirin/tylenol or anti-inflammatory drugs

5. How long have you had this pain? ☒ years ❑ months ❑ weeks
   How long have you had similar pain? ❑ years ❑ months ❑ weeks
   A. Just prior to this onset, were you completely free of symptoms? ❑ yes ☒ no
   B. Have you had any treatment for this current problem? ☒ yes ❑ no
   C. Have the treatments helped? ☒ yes ❑ no
   D. What medications are you presently taking? _None_
   E. Do you have a respiratory infection? (pneumonia, lung, sinus, cold, or cough) _None_
   F. Does your job entail long hours on your feet? ❑ yes ☒ no
   G. Does sitting with your legs crossed make this pain worse? ❑ yes ☒ no
   If yes, ❑ right leg over left? ❑ or left leg over right?
   H. Is pain worse when going ❑ up stairs, ❑ down stairs, ❑ or level ground ?
   I. Is your back pain less if you place one leg on a stool? If yes, which leg? ❑ left ❑ right
   J. Is one arm or leg colder than the other? If yes, which one? ❑ left arm ❑ right arm ❑ left leg ❑ right leg
   K. Do you have to get up frequently at night to move about and then return to bed? _No_
   Or do you find a comfortable position and then not move for fear of increasing the pain? _No_
   L. Any other comments: _____

PREVIOUS HISTORY

6. Have you had any of these diagnostic studies?

Diagnostic x-rays?	❑ yes	❑ no	date ____
CT (computes tomography) scan	❑ yes	❑ no	date ____
myelogram (x-ray with dye injection)	❑ yes	❑ no	date ____
Electromyogram (EMG)	❑ yes	❑ no	date ____
Discogram	❑ yes	❑ no	date ____
MRI (magnetic resonance imaging)	❑ yes	❑ no	date ____
Arthrogram or Sonogram	❑ yes	❑ no	date ____
Injections	❑ yes	❑ no	date ____

7. A. Have you had anything similar before this present problem? ☒ yes ❑ no
   If yes, how often? _TMJ_
   B. Are they increasing in ☒ frequency or ☒ severity?
   If yes, explain _Headaches happen 2-3 x's a week, last year only 1 x a week. Now I must go to bed when I have one. — Then could often work and continue life._

8.   A.   Have you been hospitalized for your pain problem?   ☐ yes   ☒ no
        If yes, number of times _____ dates _____
    B.   Have you had surgery for this problem? ☐ yes ☒ no   If yes, number of times _____ dates_____

9.   Have you been hospitalized for other medical problems? ☐ yes ☒ no
    If yes, number of times _____ dates_____ describe_____
_____

10.   What medications are you currently taking? (list all) _None_ _____
_____

11.   Do you take antacids? ☐ yes ☒ no

12.   Do you have any of the following conditions? (check all that apply)
☐ stomach problems?	☐ diabetes?	☐ arthritis?	☐ gout?
☐ sexual difficulties?	☐ cancer?	☐ heart?	☐ bowel or bladder problems?
☐ hypertension?	☐ epilepsy?	☐ weight loss?	☒ other? (please explain) _hypoglycemia + TMJ_

13.   Do you have allergies? ☐ yes ☒ no   Please list _____

14.   Do you smoke? ☐ yes ☒ no   If yes, how much? _____

15.   Do you drink alcoholic beverages? ☐ yes ☒ no   If yes, how much? _____

16.   What other doctors or health care providers have you seen for this condition? _Osteopath + Massage Therapist_

PERSONAL / FAMILY HISTORY
(Health Status at Present. If Deceased State Cause of Death)

Mother   E.S.   _Healthy_   Father Deleted   _- Healthy_

Children _with allergys_   Other_____

17.   Does any member of your family wear a heel lift? ☐ yes ☒ no   If yes, who _____

18.   Have you, or any member of your family, had thyroid problems? ☒ yes ☐ no   If yes, who _maternal grandmother_

19.   Have you, or any member of your family, had a recent sore throat? ☐ yes ☒ no

20.   Have you had a recent low grade fever? ☐ yes ☒ no

21.   Have you, or any member of your family had, or have, a history of Rheumatic Fever? ☐ yes ☒ no
    If yes, explain _____

22.   Have you, or any member of your family, had gout? ☐ yes ☒ no

23.   Have you recently been bitten by a spider or tick? ☐ yes ☒ no

24.   Have you had any recent venereal disease or possible exposure? ☐ yes ☒ no

25.   Do you still have any wisdom teeth remaining? ☐ yes ☒ no
    If Yes, which one(s) ☐ all remaining ☐ upper left remaining ☐ upper right remaining ☐ lower left remaining ☐ lower right remaining

26.   Do you have any missing teeth (other than wisdom)? ☐ yes ☒ no
    If yes, have they been replaced? ☐ yes ☐ no

27.   Have you had, or are you undergoing any orthodontic treatment? ☒ yes ☐ no
    If yes, were teeth extracted for this treatment? ☒ yes ☐ no - _baby teeth_

28.   Do you wear any retainers? ☐ yes ☒ no - _caused TMJ to act up_

29.   Do you wear dentures or partial dentures? ☐ yes ☒ no

30.   Have you had any of the following done? ☐ crowns ☐ caps ☐ bridgework

31.   A.   Do you grind your teeth? ☐ yes ☒ no
    B.   Does your jaw click or pop? ☒ yes ☐ no
    C.   Do you wear any appliances to treat either of these problems? ☐ yes ☒ no

32.   Have you had any dental treatment lately? ☐ yes ☒ no
    If yes, please explain _____

MISCELLANY

33.   Do you want a report sent to your attorney? ☐ yes ☒ no   ☐ I have no attorney.

34.   Do you have any additional information that would be helpful in understanding your condition? _I have been seen for a locked jaw at 16, chestpains, 16, and dizzy spells at 9 → No help from doctors, problems persist in one way or another._ _otherside →_

35.   Please indicate last grade completed in school. _Freshman yr. college_

36.   To be sure paperwork is filled out correctly, please check if appropriate:
    _____ on worker's compensation.
    _____ receiving disability income.
    _____ report should be sent to referring physician or family physician.
    _____ legal proceeding pending.
    _____ report should be sent to another party. (list name & address below)

Name:_____ E.S. _____

Address:_____

51

For the dizzy spells I had EKGs + EEG's with normal E.S.
results, they were diagnosed as hormonal. My period started at
13.

For the locked jaw I saw several different docters, was told
I didn't breath at Bethesada Naval Hospital, thats why it was
locked. The jaw unlocked ~~partially~~ after my braces were removed mid treatment.
It unlocked completly 1 year later. No pain in jaw.

For the chest pains I had an EEG and blood work done, no
results. Diagnosed as inflamed cartelege at the joints. Sometimes,
every month or two I take IB profen.

HEALTHSOUTH
Diagnostic Center of Knoxville
601 Hall of Fame Dr.
Knoxville, TN 37915

865-525-7100 Business Office
865-525-7000 Scheduling
865-525-7797 Medical Records

Account #: 141198   Our Courier

Name: STOUGH, SARA

Home Phone: (865)524-5090
Work Phone: (865)000-0000 Ext.:   0

Date of Birth: 7/28/83 Sex: F

Ref: 01678 JAMES CARLSON

Date of Procedure: 10/10/02

STANDING PELVIC RADIOGRAPHS:

Two views of the pelvis were obtained in the standing position. There are
no bony or soft tissue abnormalities. Specifically, there are no fractures
or osseous lesions.

IMPRESSION:

1. Negative study.

GLENN E. JUNG, M.D./nr

53

E.S.

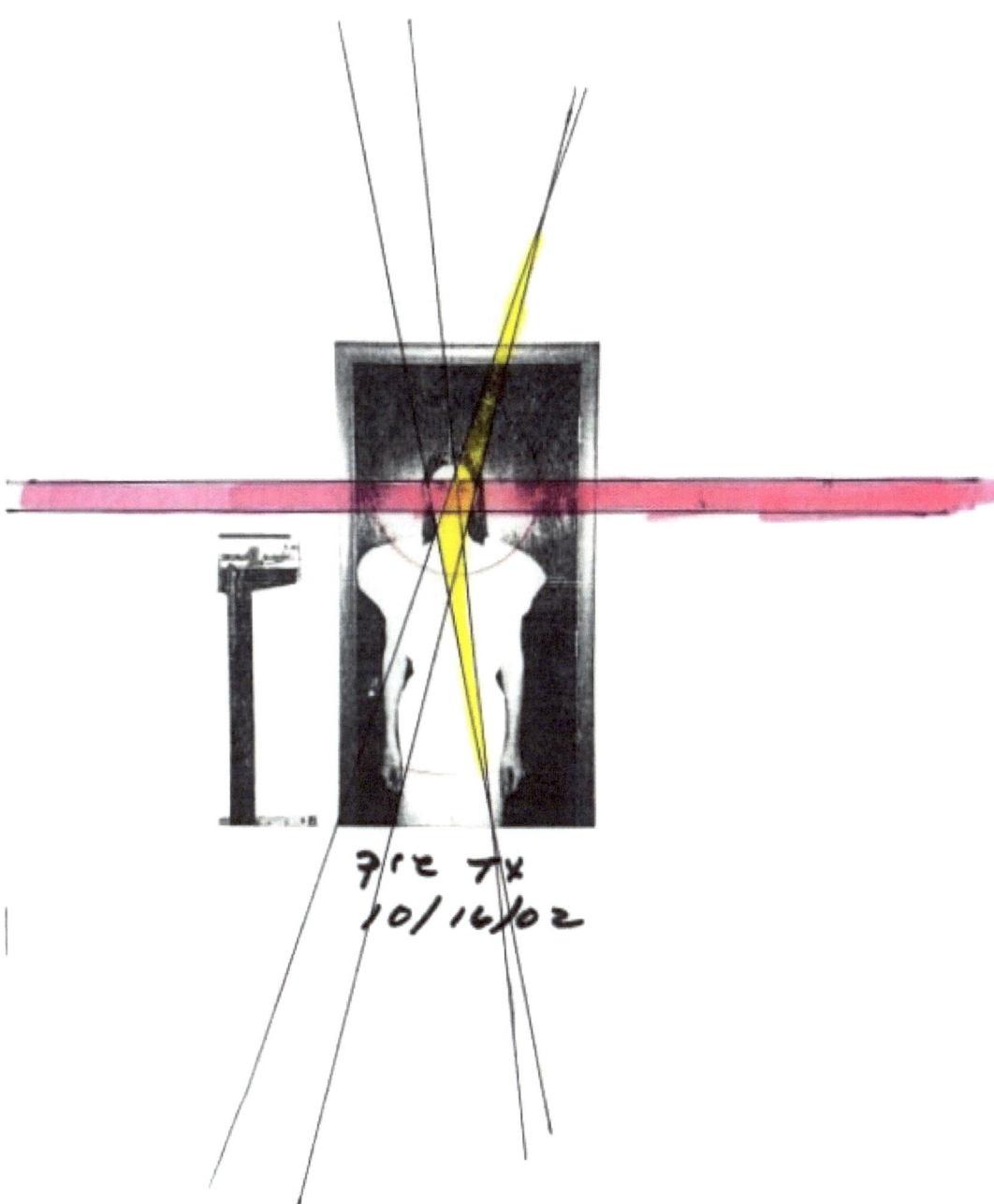

E.S.

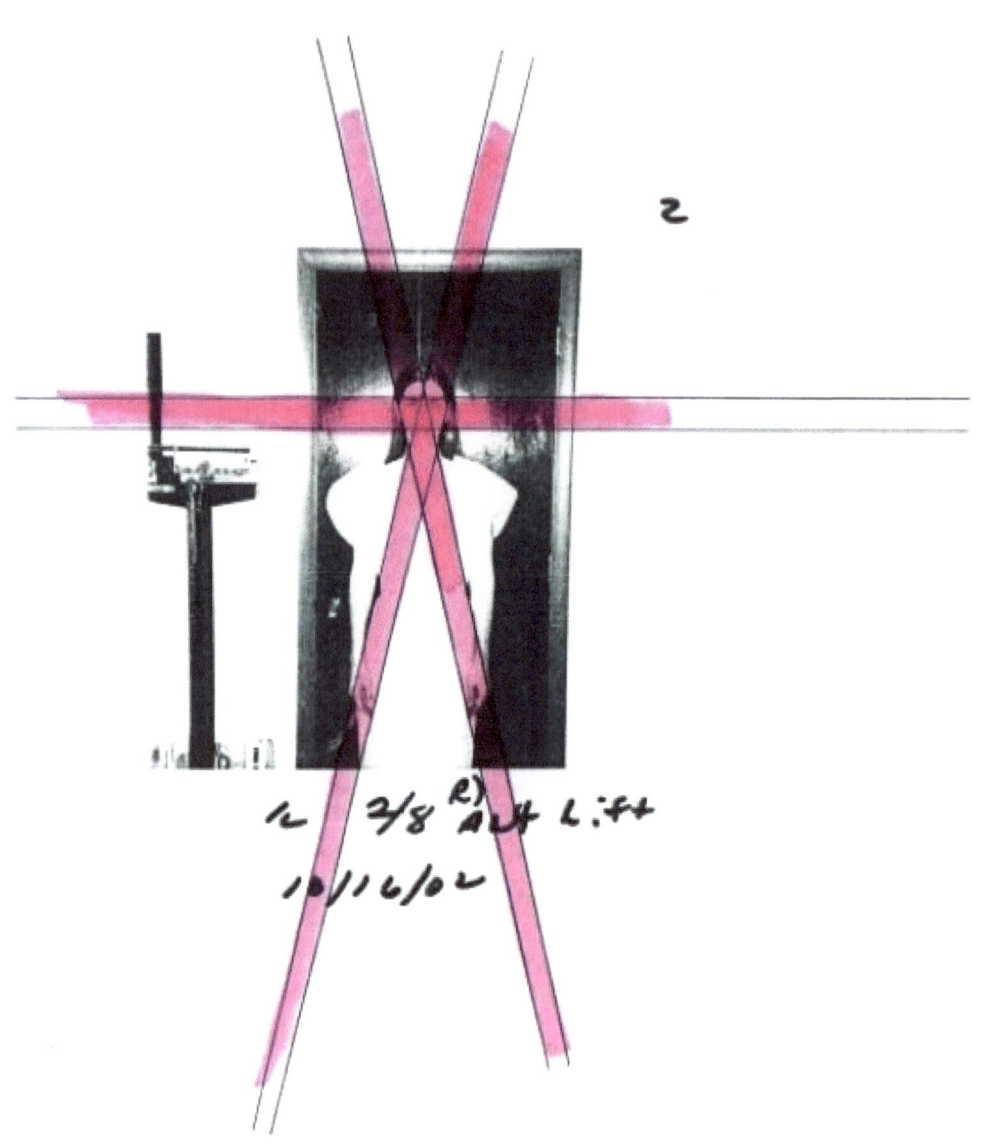

E.S.   10/16/02

This is a 19-year-old Caucasian female. She is an architecture student at the University of Tennessee. She is from Maryland. Her father was a career military individual. This is in addition to the nurses notes and the patient's filled in history. The patient brought with her AP and lateral standing pelvic x-ray. Her x-ray shows that she has an unusually long, crooked coccyx and it shows that she has some pubic symphysis abnormality as well as a spur on the left superior portion of the symphysis. She has an inferior subluxation of the symphysis.   JAC:pb

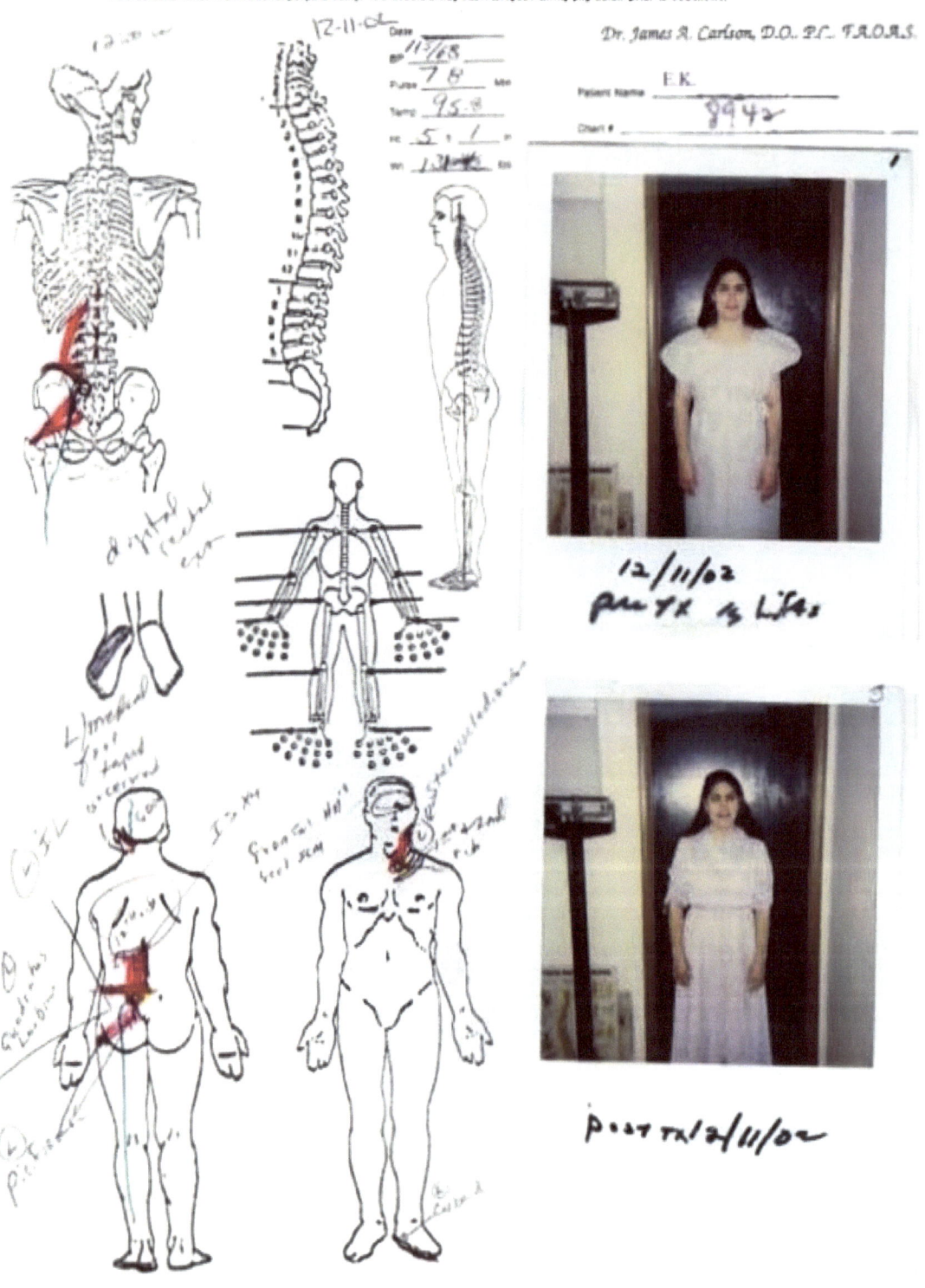

57

E.K.   2

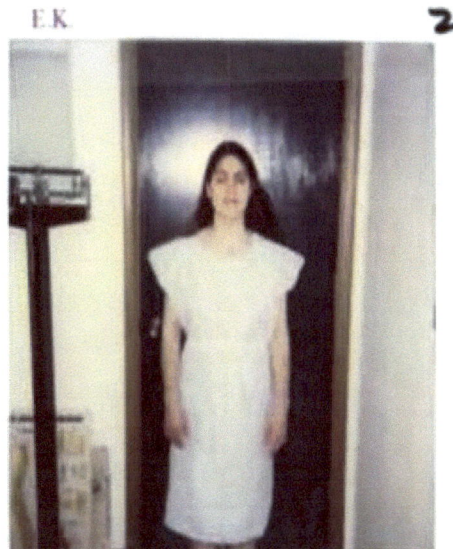

POST TX
12/ OH/02

58

James A. Carlson D.O.P.C.

PATIENT E.K.	CHART # 8942	PAGE
DATE 12-4-02 PROGRESS		PLANS

Ribs on the (L) side will not stay
in the bod this tx. + where will not
H/As 2 time per week in the afternoon
evening.
H/A more in the forehead
Pt lKs in the bak...
the had some constipation

① omt comp &
C&s/m FR
② spend
cranial tut
& Cr/m FR
③ Diag Phts
④ one day
for my site
⑤ L/ medul
for tapul
⑥ cold packs
applied to
post inj site
⑦ digital rectal
exam

E.K.

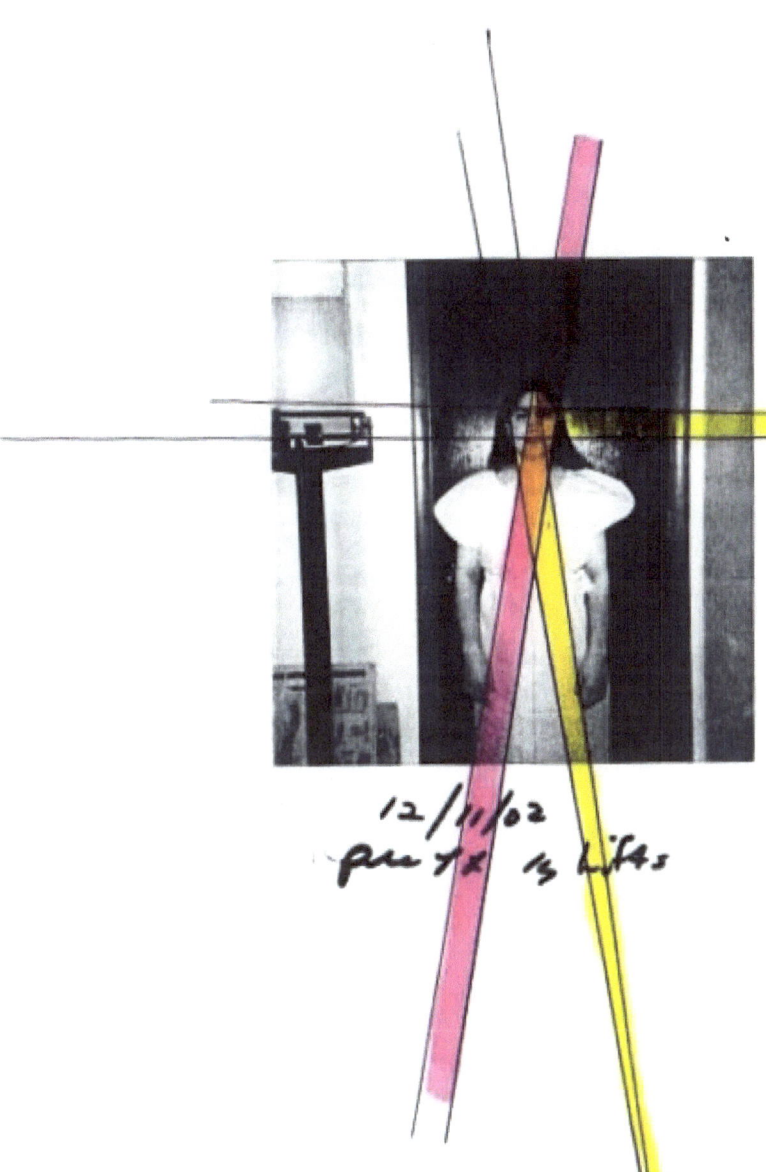

12/11/02
pre tx 1/3 lifts

E.K.

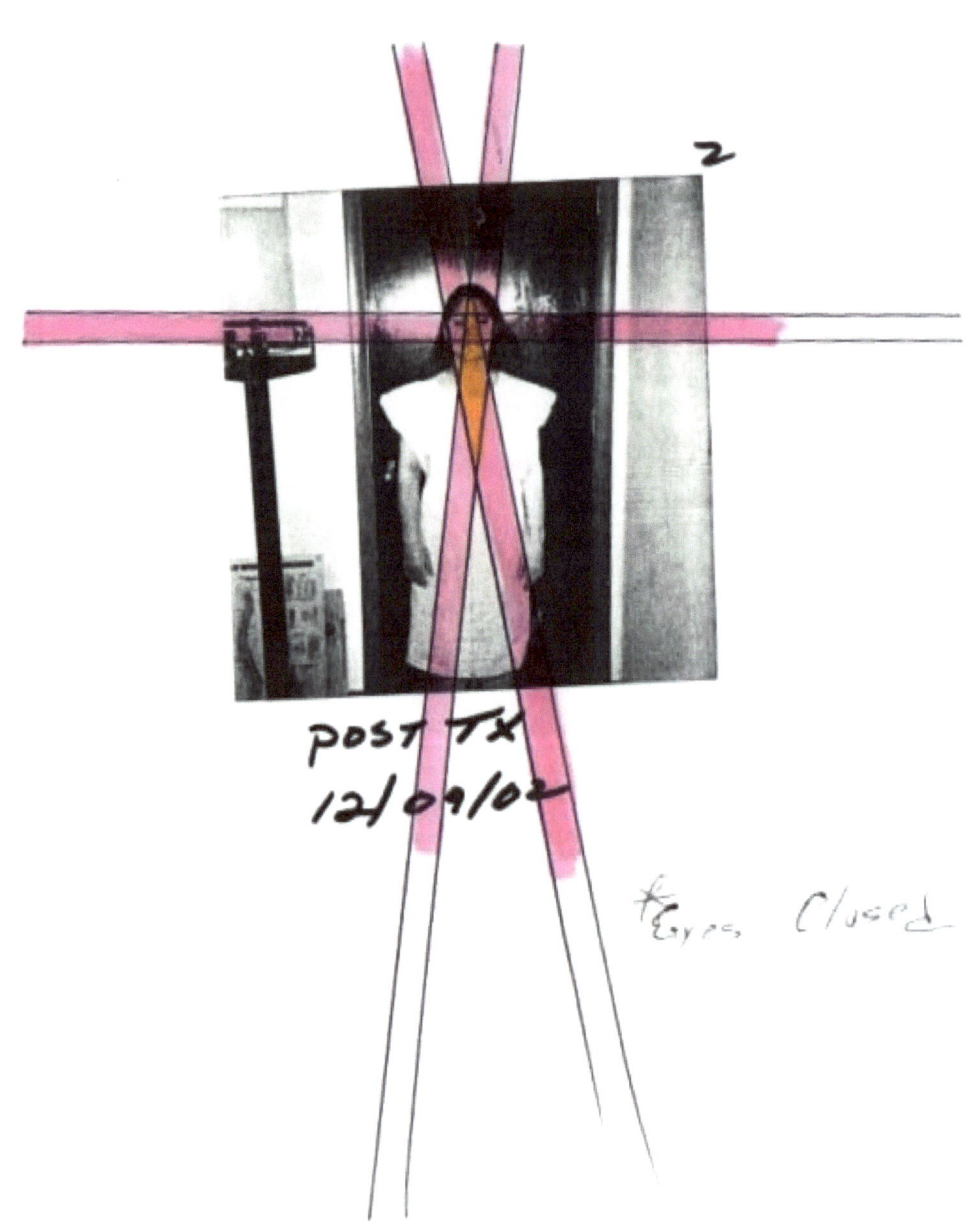

POST TX
12/09/02

*Eyes Closed

E.K.

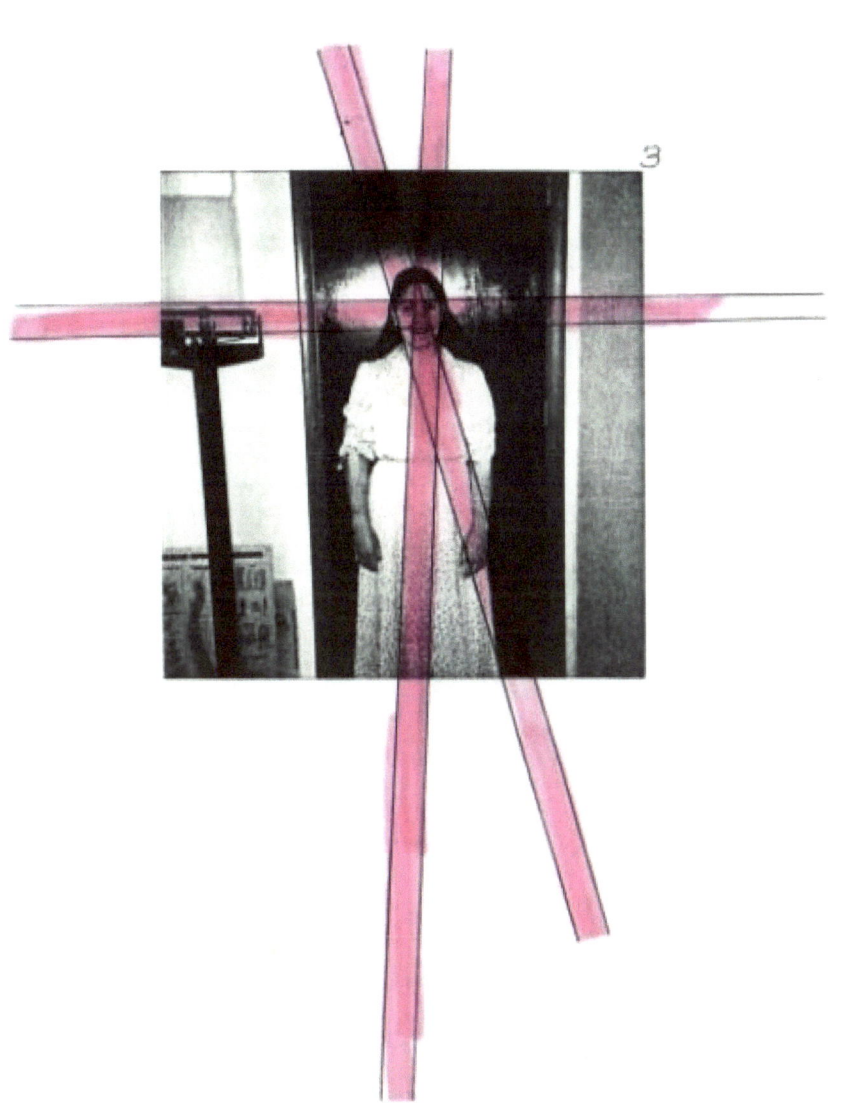

E.K.   12/11/02

She returns today with complaints of rib pain particularly. She also has some pain in the left side and has been having headaches about two times a week and she describes her headaches as being in the frontal area of her head. She has been in the bakery for several weeks now and it seems like some of these problems have reappeared. She had been doing quite well. She complains of some constipation. Examination notes that she has left piriformis involvement giving her some sciatic and radicular pain. She has tenderness at the facet joint and also at the iliolumbar ligament area on the ileum and she has quadrata laborum spasm as well as piriformis spasm and some instability of the supraspinous and interspinous ligaments of the dorsolumbar junction area. She also has second cervical involvement with greater occipital nerve entrapment. She has a first cervical subluxation. She has a left first rib and clavicle involvement. Injections were done as shown on the figure on the front page. Taping of the right foot medially to offset a navicular problem of the foot was done. I injected the foot with local anesthetic around the navicular in order to reduce the subluxation which prevented the patient from going into full extension and full flexion of the foot. She is to remove the tape tomorrow. Cold packs were applied to the injection sites postinjection. Total mobilization of the craniosacral, visceral and musculoskeletal and rectal examination were done to mobilize the bladder on the symphysis as well as to help palpate for piriformis spasm. Posttreatment the patient is parallel in three dimensions but she still has a symmetrical deviation. The patient was told to remove the tape tomorrow and use cold packs to the injection sites p.r.n. and drink copious amounts of water for the next few days. She is to avoid heavy lifting particularly for the next week. She has a set of exercises given a friend by a chiropractor which were stretching exercises and I see no reason why she cannot perform these particularly since she had been before and was doing well.   JAC:pb

Initial visit photo contrast to final photo

E.K.

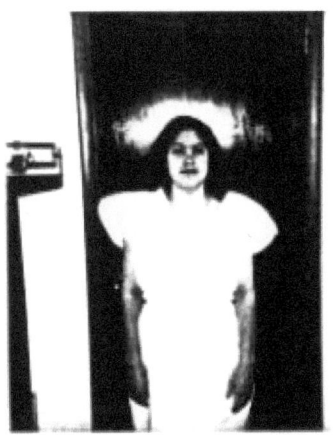

11/28/00
is shoes pre TX

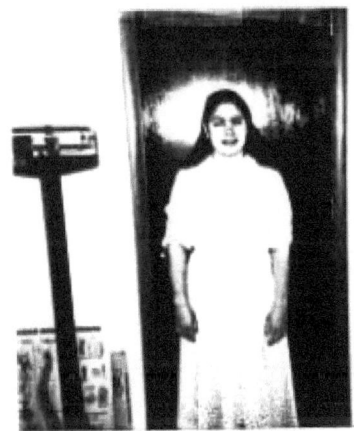

Post TX 2/11/02

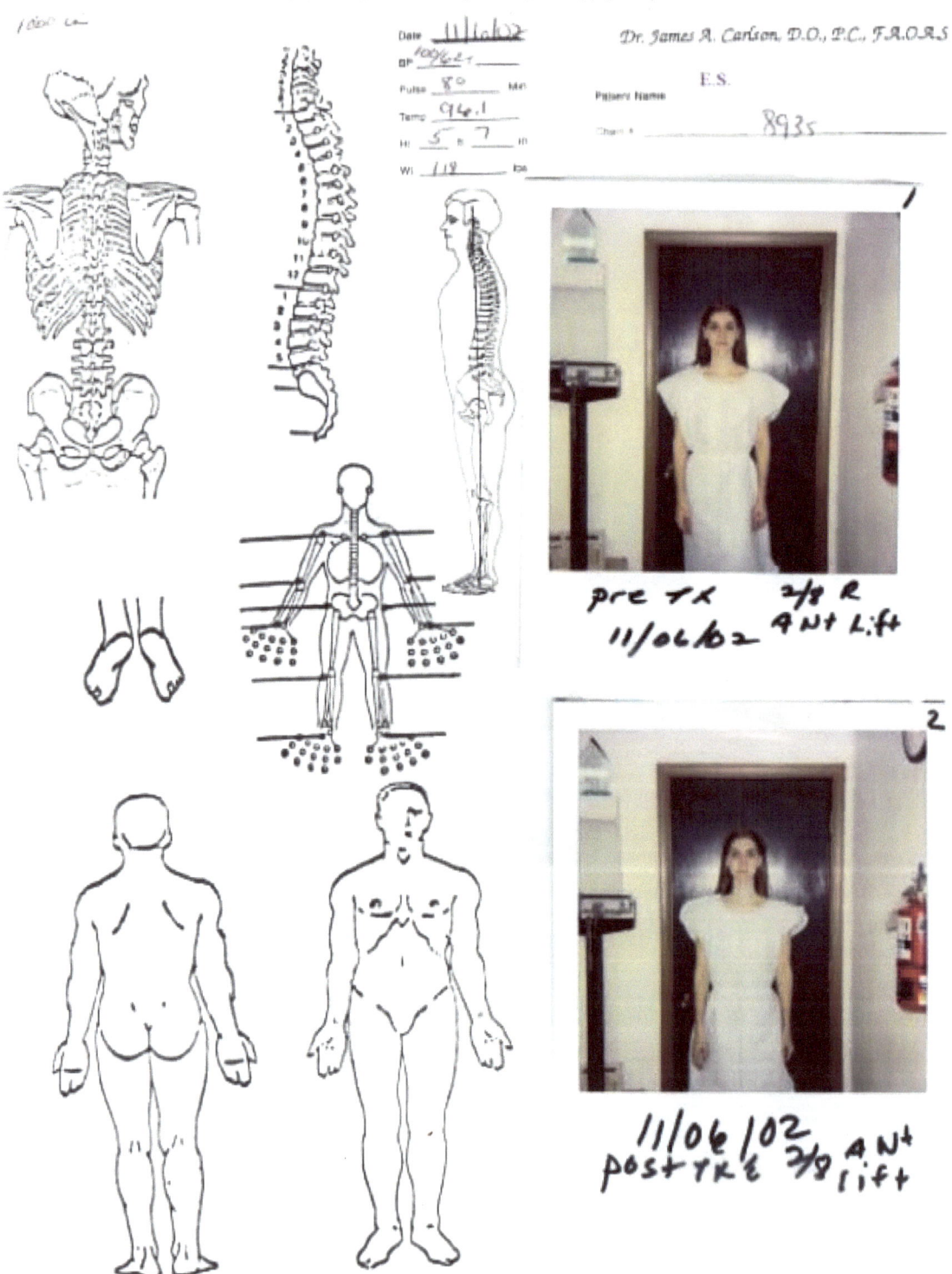

Date 11/06/02
BP 100/62T
Pulse 80 Min
Temp 96.1
Ht 5 7 in
Wt 118 lbs

Dr. James A. Carlson, D.O., P.C., F.A.O.A.S

E.S.
Patient Name

Chart # 8935

pre TX 3/8 R
11/06/02 ANt Lift

11/06/02
POSt TXE 3/8 ANt lift

James A. Carlson D.O.P.C.

PATIENT E.S.	CHART # 8935	PAGE
DATE 11/6/02 PROGRESS		PLANS

Has had 3 H/A a less severness. Can now
feel baromete change in ear thu has come
back. Noticed this @ the age of 16 in the
beginning when jaw 1st locked.

Has noticed NO MORE hip clicking

Pt did discuss this tx c her mother
t that there is ok if more is needed

(1) OMT complete
c Cos/mfr
(2) Special cranial
tech c Cos/mfr
(3) Diag Photos
(4)

Pt is to continue
wearing her lift
R 3/8 Ant. Lift

E.S.

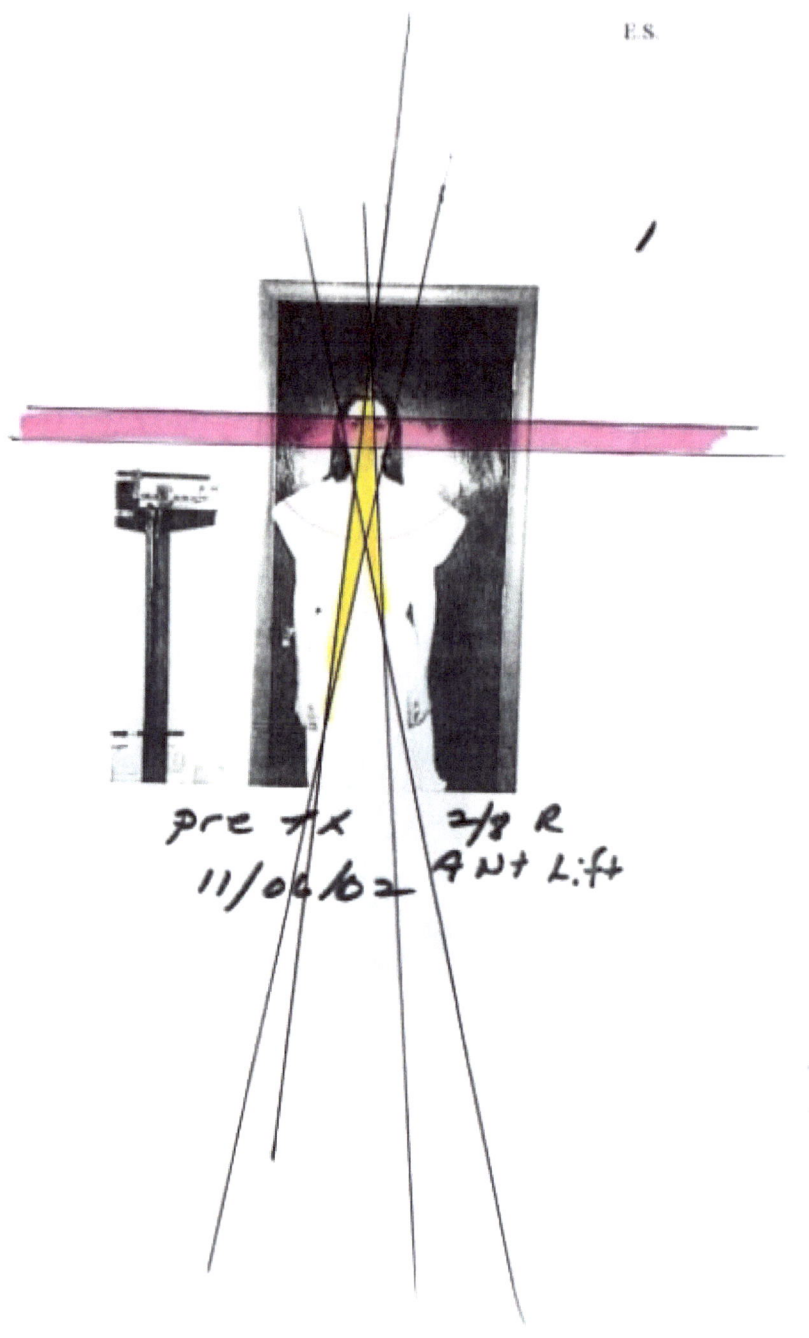

pre tx   2/8 R
11/06/62   Ant Lift

E.S.

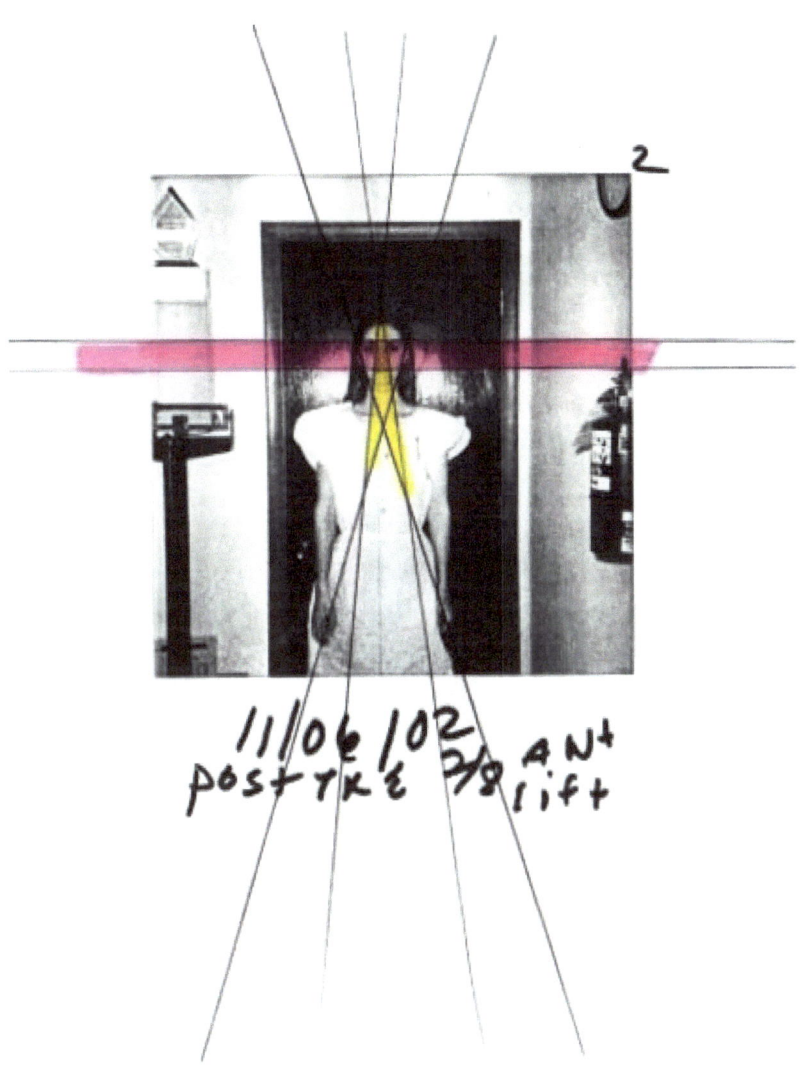

11/06/02
posture ANt
3/8 lift

E.S.

11/06/02

She returns today. She is improved. She has had less headaches. She has had less clicking in her TMJ's and the clicking in her hip no longer happens. I discussed this with her mother and her mother agrees that sclerotherapy would probably be helpful to her. However, I feel that she is doing well enough at this point that mobilization is all that she needs at this time. I did do total mobilization of the craniosacral, visceral and musculoskeletal. I have asked her to return if she has anymore problems. If she continues to have the same problem we would consider sclerotherapy.   JAC:pb

PATIENT PAIN DRAWING

Name W.H. _____ Date _____

Mark the areas on your body where you feel the sensations decribed below, using the appropriate symbol. Mark the areas of radiation. Include all affected areas.

Aching	Numbness	Pins and needles	Burning	Stabbing
▲▲▲	---	000	xxx	///

Please mark with an X, on the drawing above, at the location where the pain is worst now. How bad is your pain now? Please mark on the line below how bad your pain is now.

No pain <-----|-----|-----|-----|-----|-----|-----|-----|-----|-----|-----|-----|-----|----->Worst possible pain

8. A. Have you been hospitalized for your pain problem? ☐ yes ☑ no
    If yes, number of times _____ dates _____
    B. Have you had surgery for this problem? ☐ yes ☑ no   If yes, number of times _____ dates_____
9. Have you been hospitalized for other medical problems? ☑ yes ☐ no
    If yes, number of times _____ dates _1951_ describe_____
    _____ *appendectomy*_____
10. What medications are you currently taking? (list all)
    _____ *none – except Evista for bones*_____
11. Do you take antacids? ☐ yes   ☑ no
12. Do you have any of the following conditions? (check all that apply)
    ☐ stomach problems?   ☐ diabetes?   ☐ arthritis?   ☐ gout?
    ☐ sexual difficulties?   ☐ cancer?   ☐ heart?   ☐ bowel or bladder problems?
    ☐ hypertension?   ☐ epilepsy?   ☐ weight loss?   ☐ other? (please explain)_____
13. Do you have allergies? ☑ yes ☐ no   Please list _*lactose*_____
14. Do you smoke? ☐ yes   ☑ no If yes, how much?_____
15. Do you drink alcoholic beverages? ☑ yes   ☐ no   If yes, how much? *occasional glass of wine*
16. What other doctors or health care providers have you seen for this condition? *Dr. Berry (chiropractor)*

PERSONAL / FAMILY HISTORY
(Health Status at Present. If Deceased State Cause of Death)

Mother *Clara Cogdill (heart)*   Father *Hobart Cogdill (lung cancer)*
Children *5*   Other_____

17. Does any member of your family wear a heel lift? ☐ yes ☑ no If yes, who_____
18. Have you, or any member of your family, had thyroid problems? ☐ yes ☑ no If yes, who_____
19. Have you, or any member of your family, had a recent sore throat? ☐ yes ☑ no
20. Have you had a recent low grade fever? ☐ yes ☑ no
21. Have you, or any member of your family had, or have, a history of Rheumatic Fever? ☐ yes ☑ no
    If yes, explain _____
22. Have you, or any member of your family, had gout? ☐ yes ☑ no
23. Have you recently been bitten by a spider or tick? ☐ yes ☑ no
24. Have you had any recent venereal disease or possible exposure? ☐ yes ☑ no
25. Do you still have any wisdom teeth remaining? ☑ yes ☐ no
    If Yes, which one(s) ☐ all remaining ☑ upper left remaining ☐ upper right remaining ☐ lower left remaining ☐ lower right remaining
26. Do you have any missing teeth (other than wisdom)? ☑ yes ☐ no
    If yes, have they been replaced? ☑ yes ☐ no
27. Have you had, or are you undergoing any orthodontic treatment? ☐ yes ☑ no
    If yes, were teeth extracted for this treatment? ☐ yes ☐ no
28. Do you wear any retainers? ☐ yes ☑ no
29. Do you wear dentures or partial dentures? ☑ yes ☐ no
30. Have you had any of the following done? ☑ crowns ☐ caps ☐ bridgework
31. A. Do you grind your teeth? ☐ yes ☑ no
    B. Does your jaw click or pop? ☐ yes ☑ no
    C. Do you wear any appliances to treat either of these problems? ☐ yes ☑ no
32. Have you had any dental treatment lately? ☑ yes ☐ no
    If yes, please explain *Routine cleaning + checkup*

MISCELLANY

33. Do you want a report sent to your attorney? ☐ yes ☑ no ☐ I have no attorney.
34. Do you have any additional information that would be helpful in understanding your condition? *No*
35. Please indicate last grade completed in school. *post graduate college (MA)*
36. To be sure paperwork is filled out correctly, please check if appropriate:
    _____ on worker's compensation.
    _____ receiving disability income.
    _____ report should be sent to referring physician or family physician.
    _____ legal proceeding pending.
    _____ report should be sent to another party. (list name & address below)
Name: _*W.H.*_____
Address:_____

W.H

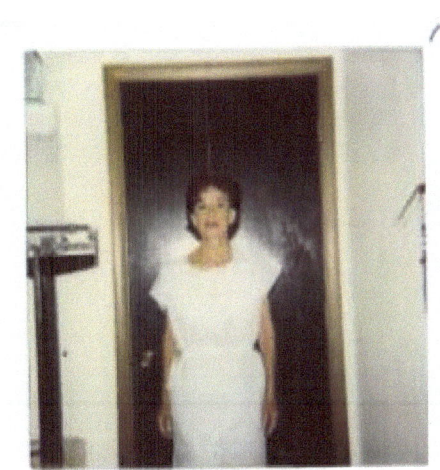

Pre TX
5/30/03

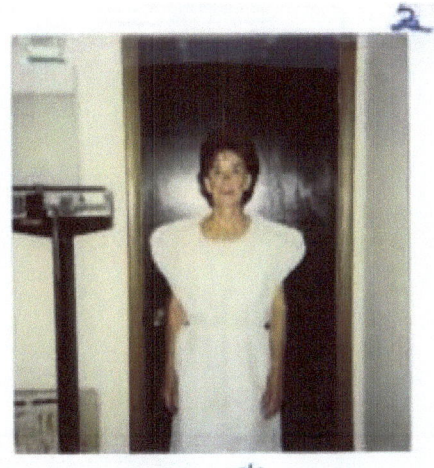

POST TX
5/30/03

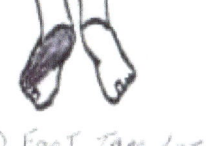

① FOOT Tape Lat.

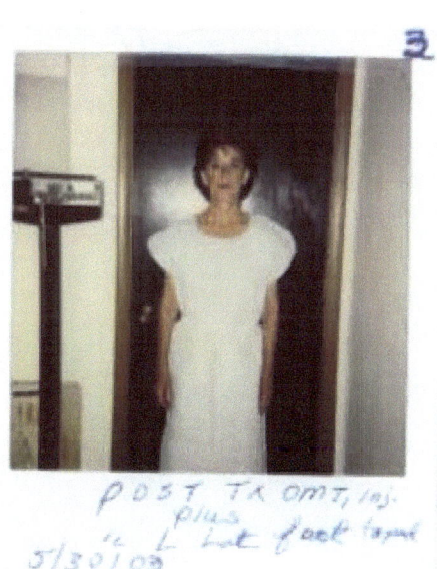

POST TR OMT, inj.
plus
" L Lat foot tape
5/30/03

Date 5/30/03

BP 120/68

Pulse 78 Min

Temp 97.5

Ht 5 ft 7 in

Wt 116 lbs

Dr. James A. Carlson, D.O., P.C., F.A.O.A.S.

Patient Name W.H.

Chart # 8958

* Needs ® Gluteal Lift.

James A. Carlson D.O.P.C.

PATIENT Wilma Haggard   CHART # 8958   PAGE

DATE 5/30/03 PROGRESS   PLANS

Retired from school administrator
Worked in Saudi Arabia 24yrs raised 5 children
husband - orthodonist

Back pain past 3-4yrs.
S. Having trouble patient c̄ (back problems)first noticed
Pt goes to Dr Berry (Chiro) @ times

Pt has a full upper denture (has worn this upper 1yr)
Has 1 down left 3rd molar which is attached to the bridge

PLANS

1. New Pt History
2. Review X-Rays
3. Established pt sitting position see diagram
4. Sublaxed coccyx w/
5. ↑ tenderness in the coccyx
6. OMT Corp c̄ C/S /MFR
7. special cranial techs C/S /MFR
8. Diag Photos x2
9. Digital rectal exam
   & located coccyx
10. (L) Lat foot (illeg)
11. Pt did read school/ProBiz ... ...
12. To RTC 2wks
   Pt advised to use cold packs & no stimulat-

→ Pt is to make a
pillow to sit on
for (R) buttock

74

Dr. James A. Carlson, D.O., P.C., F.A.O.A.S.

509 N. Cedar Bluff Rd. • Knoxville, Tennessee 37923

Name _Wilma Haggard_   Patient _8958_   Date _5/30/03_

Scar (approximate weight at time of scar) _____ lbs. _____ date

Billfold: ❑ (Right)	or ❑ (Left) Hip	Bra ❑	Hat ❑	Belt ❑
Hair Piece ❑	Hair up tight ❑	Rings: ❑ (Right)	or ❑ (Left)	or ❑ (Both)
Shoe Lifts ❑	High Heels ❑	Dentures ❑	Braces ❑	Bridges ❑
Wrist Watch: ❑ (Right)	or ❑ (Left) handed	Glasses: ❑ Full Time	❑ Part Time	Last Eye Exam _____

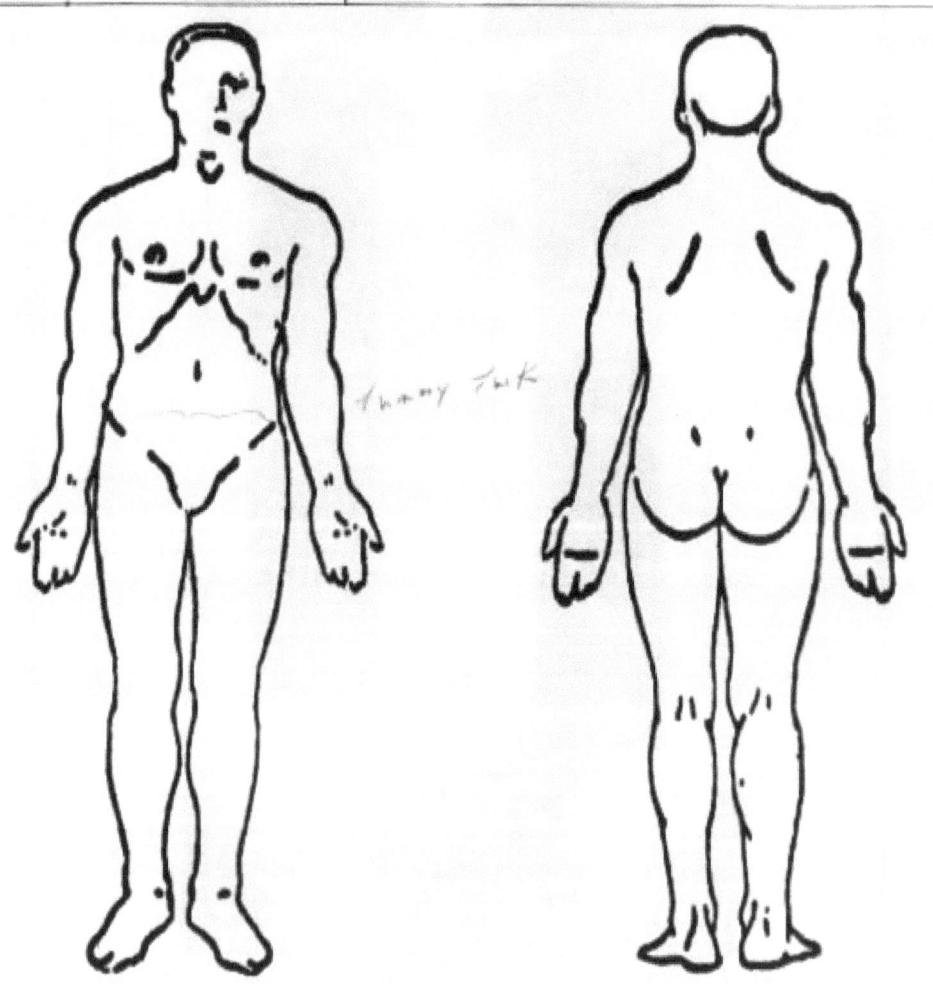

What are your expectations of your visit with Dr Carlson today? _____

75

W.H.

05/30/03

INITIAL VISIT. This is a 72-year-old Caucasian female who is retired. Her husband is a retired orthodontist. They have lived in Saudi Arabia for years and years and are back home now living in Sevierville. She notes that she has low back pain and it is only when she is sitting. She notes this has probably been a big problem at least for the last four months. Her standing AP and lateral pelvic x-ray shows what appears to be inflammation around L5. She does have a slight left pelvic depression when she is standing and has some mild anterior rotation of the left ilium. She has some early degenerative disk of the symphysis particularly at the superior pole with what appears to be possibly some early spurring at this level.

Her diagnostic photograph would show that she had a right cranial strain, some right anterior sacral problem and the left sciatic pattern. I set her on the table and she did have low back pain. I then put my hand under her right buttocks as a lift and she said the pain was not there.

I have asked her to fix her a gluteal pillow to help elevate the gluteus on the outside to see if this gives her some relief. She says that she cannot hardly sit to watch the news without leaning over to get comfortable laying down. The patient does have full upper dentures and I feel that this is a problem as well since she never takes it out day or night. I have asked her to be sure that she takes it out at night to give the bite a chance to unwind.

I did inject the interspinous ligaments at L4,5 and L5,S1 and the sacral coccyx joint which is subluxed then I sat her up again and there was really no pain at that time. She has unstable ligaments at this level including the iliolumbar ligament. These were injected with local anesthetic and proliferans solution. Total mobilization was done of the craniosacral, visceral and musculoskeletal. Rectal exam was done to reduce the coccyx and I taped the left lateral foot to relieve the sciatic strain.

Following the treatment and taping of the left lateral foot, the patient became symmetrical. I have asked her to take the tape off tomorrow and return to the clinic in two weeks for followup.
JAC:pb

WH

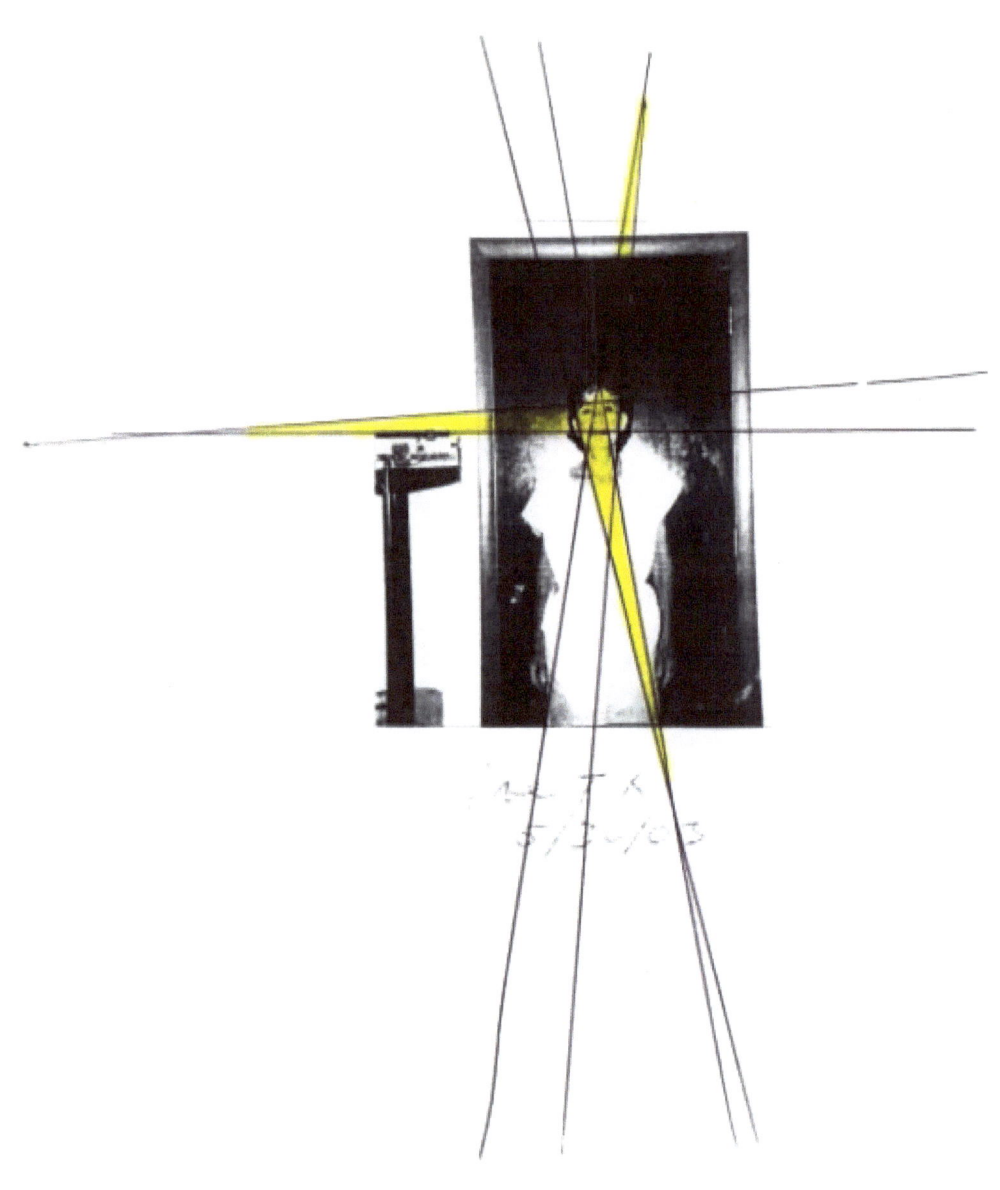

W.H.

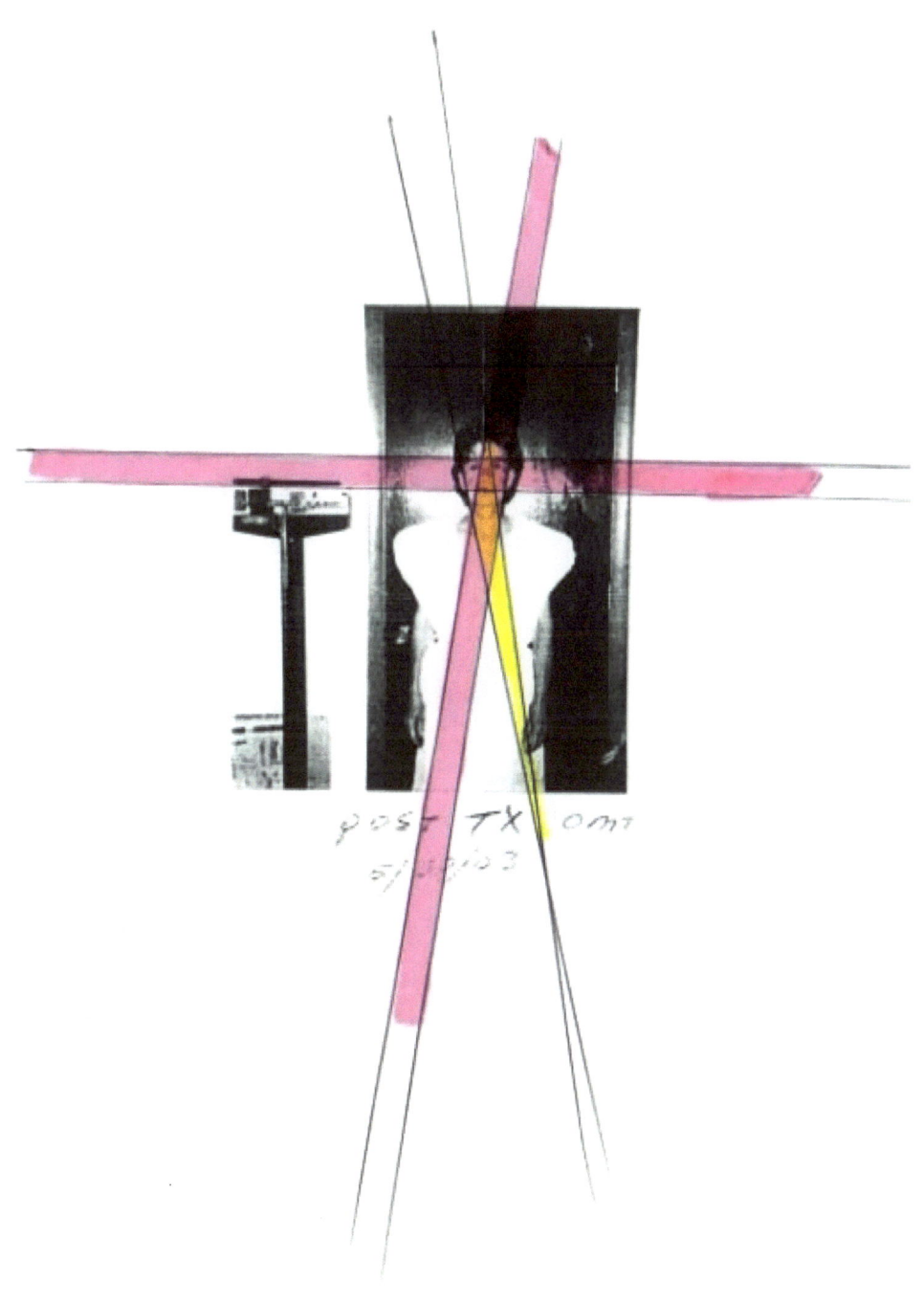

post TX oms
5/23/03

W.H.

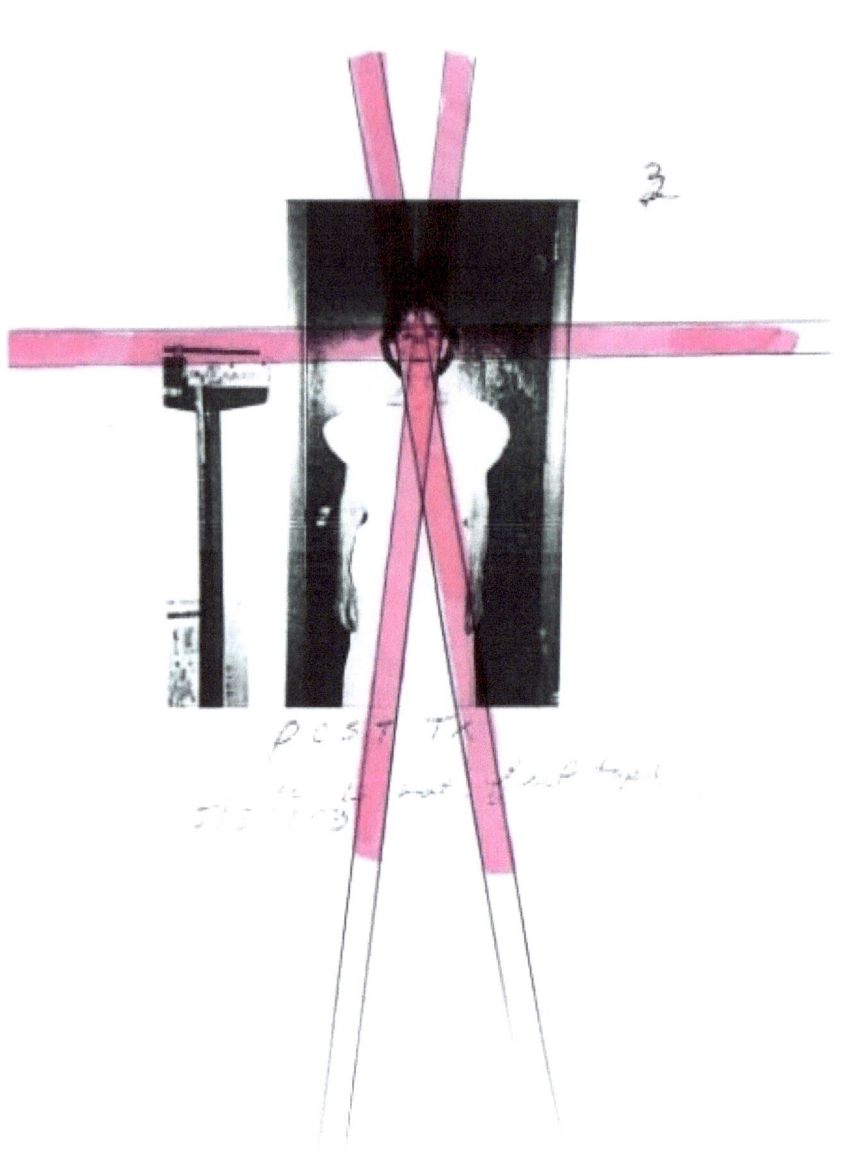

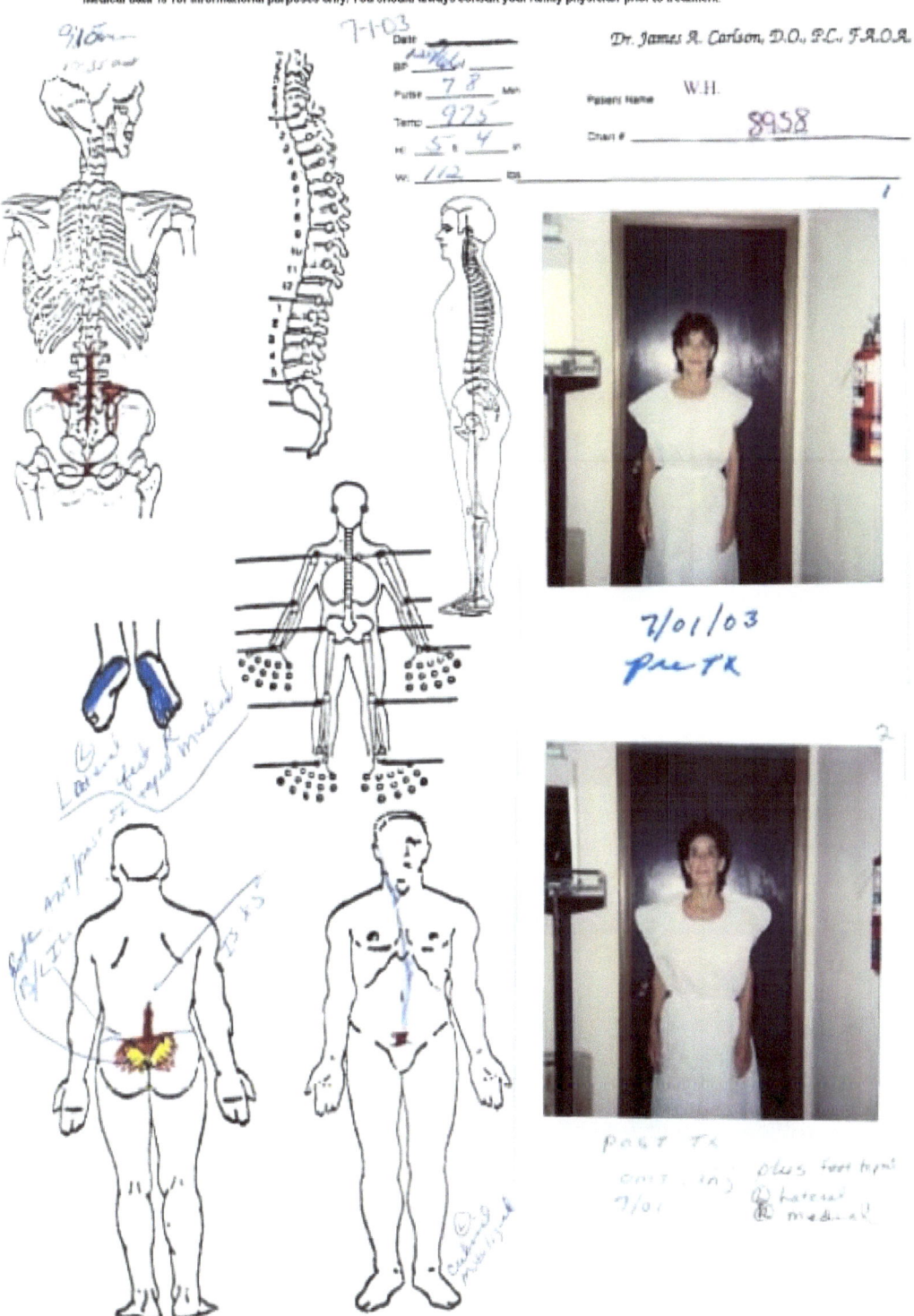

Dr. James R. Carlson, D.O., P.C., F.A.O.A.

Date _____ 7-1-03

BP _____

Pulse _____ 7 8 _____ Min

Temp _____ 97.5

Ht _____ 5' 4" _____ in

Wt _____ 112 _____ lbs

Patient Name _____ W.H.

Chart # _____ 8958

7/01/03
pre Tx

Post Tx

James A. Carlson D.O.P.C.

PATIENT	W.H.		CHART # 8958	PAGE

DATE	PROGRESS	PLANS
7-1-03	complain of center of lower back today Pt can bend over now. + was unable to before 'a.p am + he short. for 2 yrs	① OMT Comp c C5/MFR ② Special Cranial treat c C5/MFR ③ Diag Photo ④ O/L first tape ⑤ are long forms, etc ⑥

W.II.

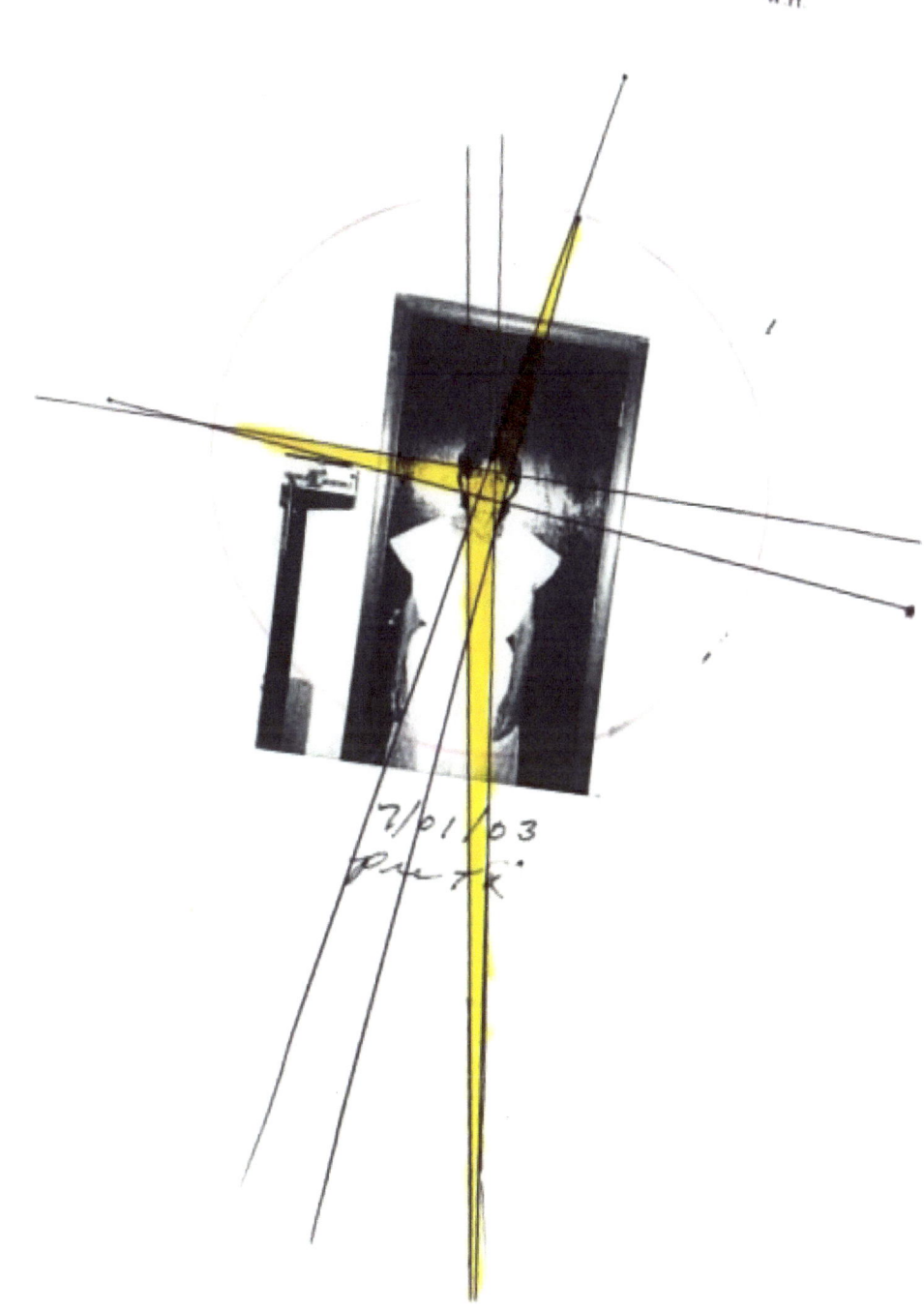

7/01/03

82

W.H.

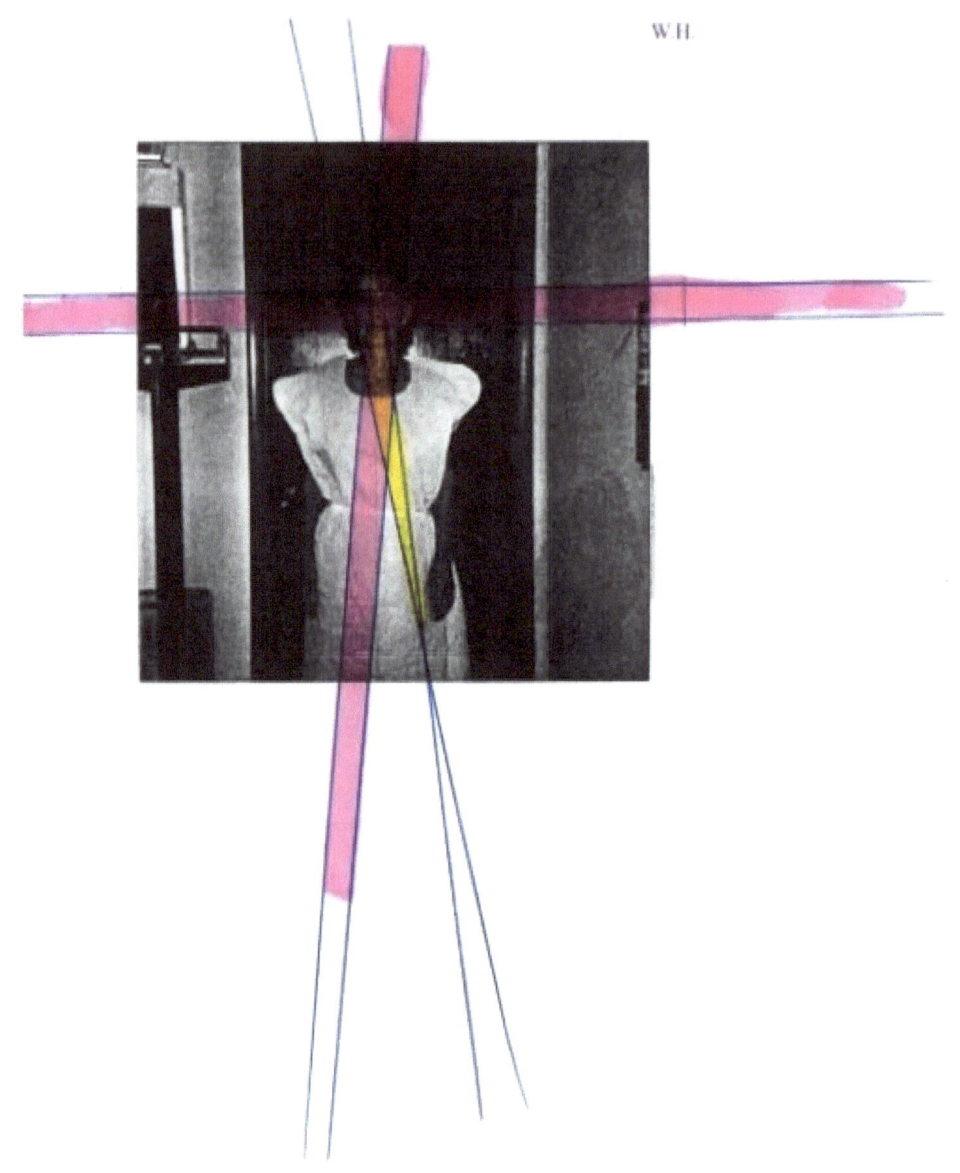

W.H. .   07/01/03

She returns today. She is thrilled. She says that for the first time that she can remember she can actually bend over and tie her shoes. She still has some pain in the center of her back and still has the instability of her pelvis but she also has an old cuboid lesion on the left foot with subluxation of the cuboid. I injected with local anesthetic around the cuboid and then the cuboid was mobilized. I repeated the sclerotherapy to the sacroiliac ligaments as well as the interspinous and supraspinous ligaments of the lower lumbar and the pubic symphysis. I did total mobilization of the extremities, pelvis, spine and cranial. She had a good cranial rhythm posttreatment. I have asked her to drink copious amounts of water and use cold packs for discomfort. We will see her again in about three weeks. I suspect that she will continue to improve and get well for us.   JAC:pb

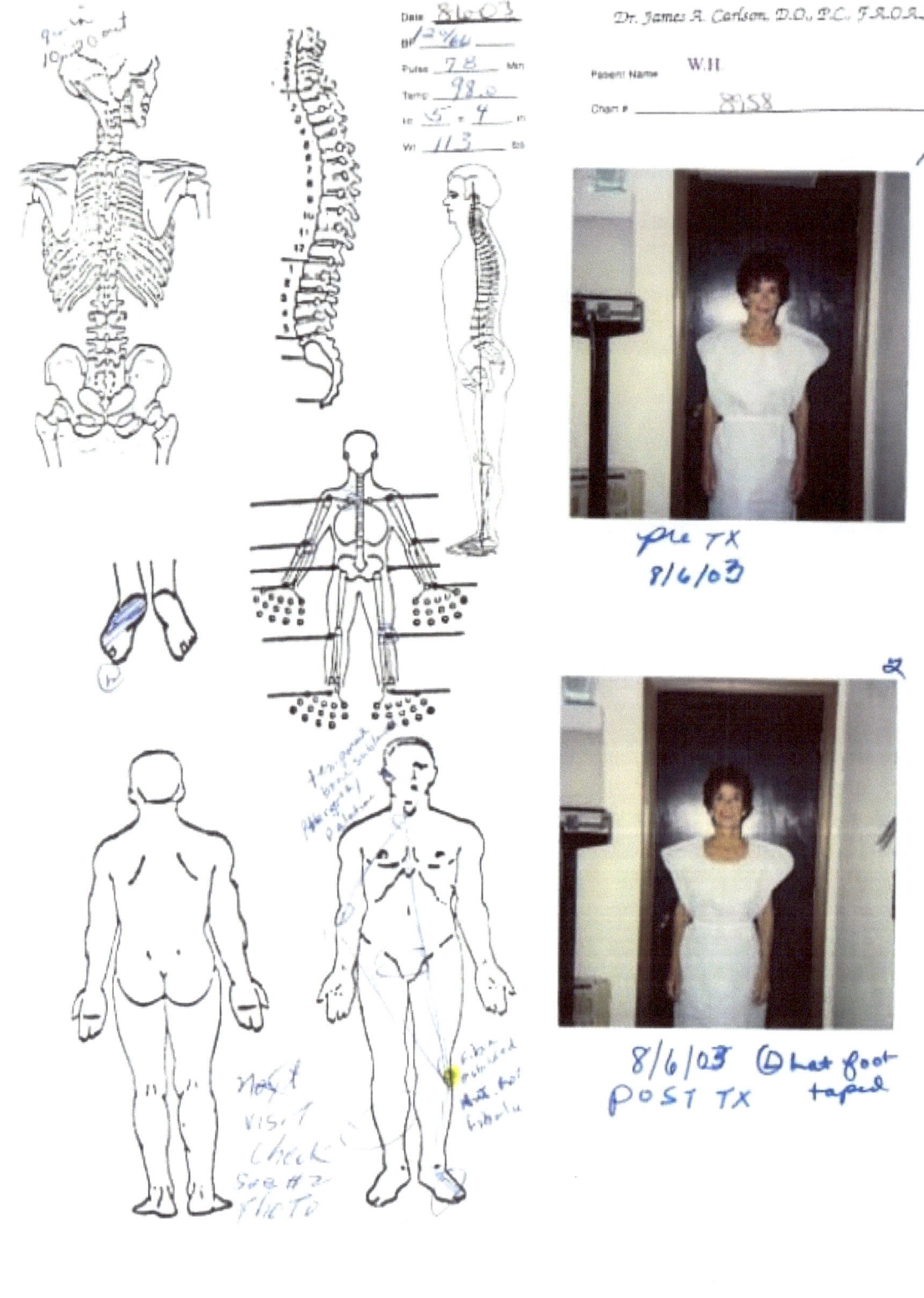

Date 8/6/03
BP 12 %66
Pulse 78 Min
Temp 98.0
ht 5 4 in
Wt 113 lbs

Dr. James A. Carlson, D.O., P.C., F.A.O.A.S.

Patient Name W.H.

Chart # 8958

pre TX
8/6/03

8/6/03 (L) Lat foot
POST TX taped

James A. Carlson D.O.P.C.

PATIENT	W.H.		CHART # 8958		PAGE

DATE	PROGRESS	PLANS
7-1-03	complain of center of lower back today	1) OMT Comp
		c C̄s/MFR
	Pt can bend over now. I was unable	2) Special
	to before 'g p.m. + tie shoes. for 2 yrs	Cranial trea
		c C̄s/MFR
		3) Diag Photo
		4) b/c foot taped
		5) see leg
		from site
		6)

Medical data is for informational purposes only. You should always consult your family physician prior to treatment.

W.H.

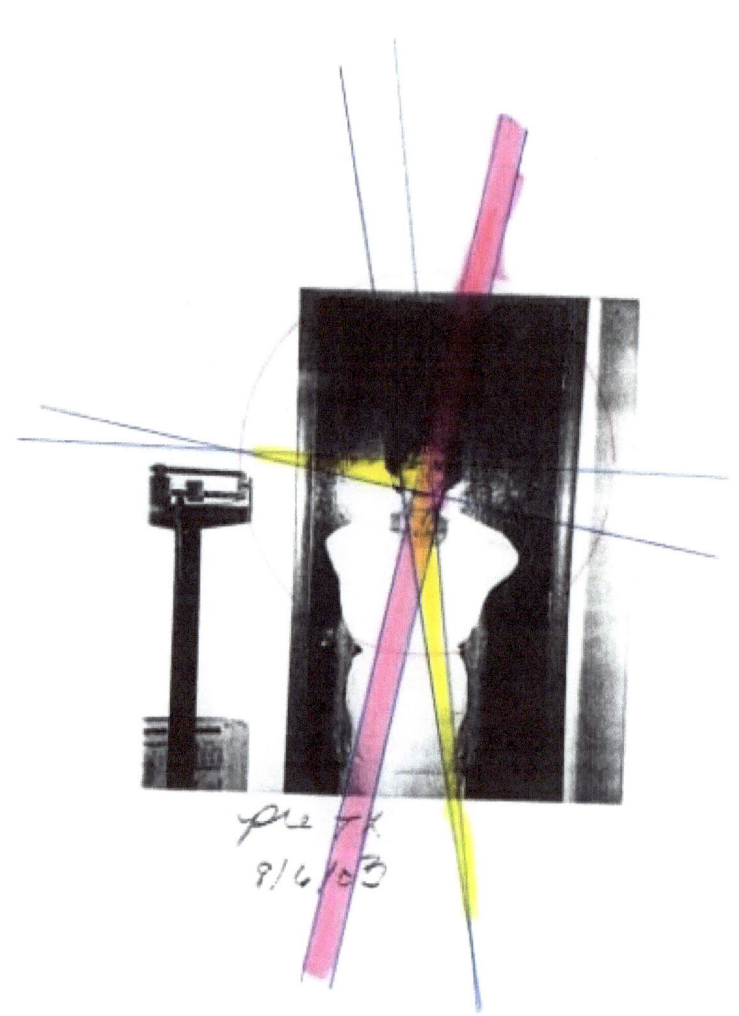

W H

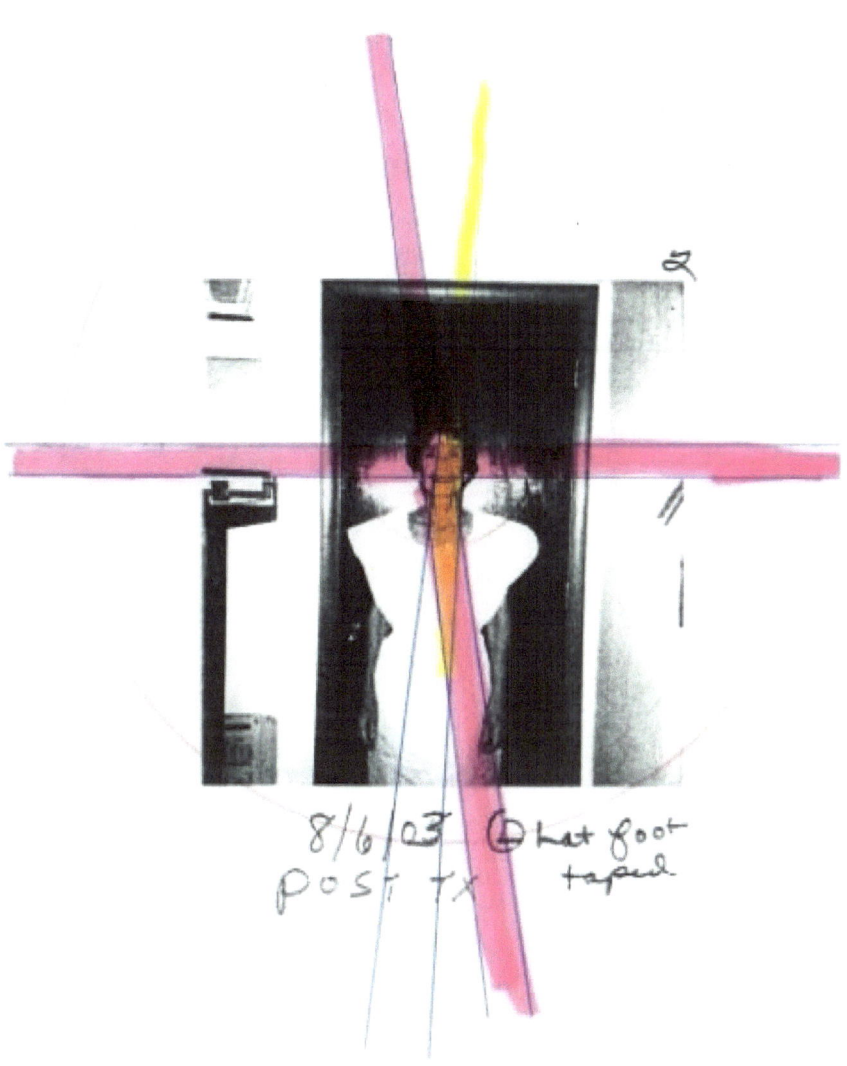

W.H.

08/06/03

She returns today. Her back still feels great. Her left foot feels tight when she flexes it. She just got back from Brazil, being a missionary.

On examination, the diagnostic photography shows that her face is certainly twisted with a temporal bone anterior on the right. Physical examination would note that the patient has a left fibular tibial proximal head anterior rotated with some tenderness along the extensor muscle as well as some of the anterior tibia. I did after trying to reduce it without local anesthetic, put local anesthetic into the fibular tibial joint and was able to rotate it back into its phase with the other one and the foot and leg pain resolved quickly. I then mobilized the opposite elbow since it is the reciprocal as well as the right clavicle. I did total mobilization of the craniosacral, visceral and musculoskeletal. I did tape the foot temporarily to help mobilize it and then I told her to remove the tape tomorrow. Posttreatment photograph would show the patient still has some right lower leg dysfunction and some symphysis dysfunction but the patient feels well at this point and I will check those the next time she returns. She is having no symptoms per se, only the hint that these are a problem on the photograph. I have asked her to return on a p.r.n. basis.   JAC:pb

Date 8-25-03

Dr. James R. Carlson, D.O., P.C., F.R.O.A.

BP ___/___

Patient Name E.S.

Pulse 80 Min

Chart # 8935

Temp 98.5

Ht 5 7 in

Wt 116 lb

's Lift
8/25/03

's Lift w/ L Lat
8/25/03   taped

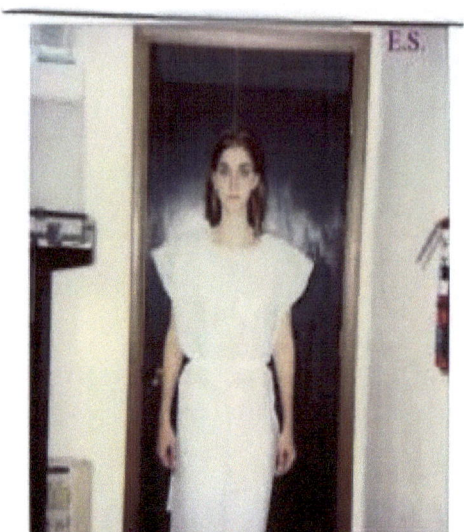

ċ ¼ ant@b.f.
8/25/07

James A. Carlson D.O.P.C.

PATIENT E.S.	CHART # 8935	PAGE
DATE 8·25·03 PROGRESS		PLANS

Chief complaint
1 time every 2 weeks migraines
Neck is cracking 20-30 times a day
Some time last semester noticed
the change in this
If pt moves neck + it cracks this will
go away 50% of time

① emt Comp
  " Ces/mre
② special
  cranial + ev.
  " Ces/mre
③ Diag Photo
④ L Lat foot + spil
⑤ Digital model exam
⑥ digital destalization
  of nessun
⑦ Dispense ② Heel
  lifts & strips
  B arches foam tape
  & extra strip also
  as pt had done
  prev. left + also
  mention au estrol

★ Post diag Photo
  Pt Does Not
  need a lift
  @ this time

92

E.S.

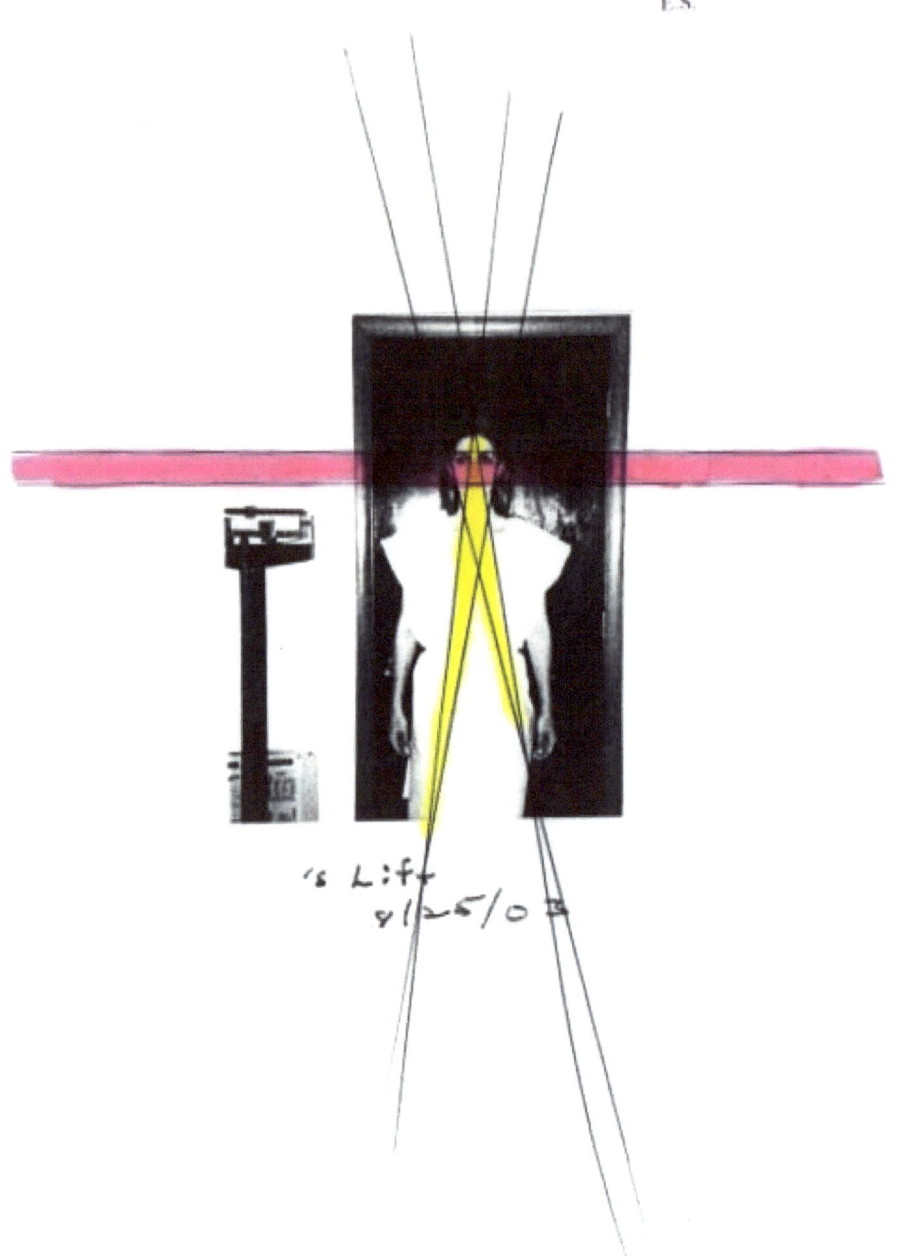

's Lift
4/25/0 B

93

E.S

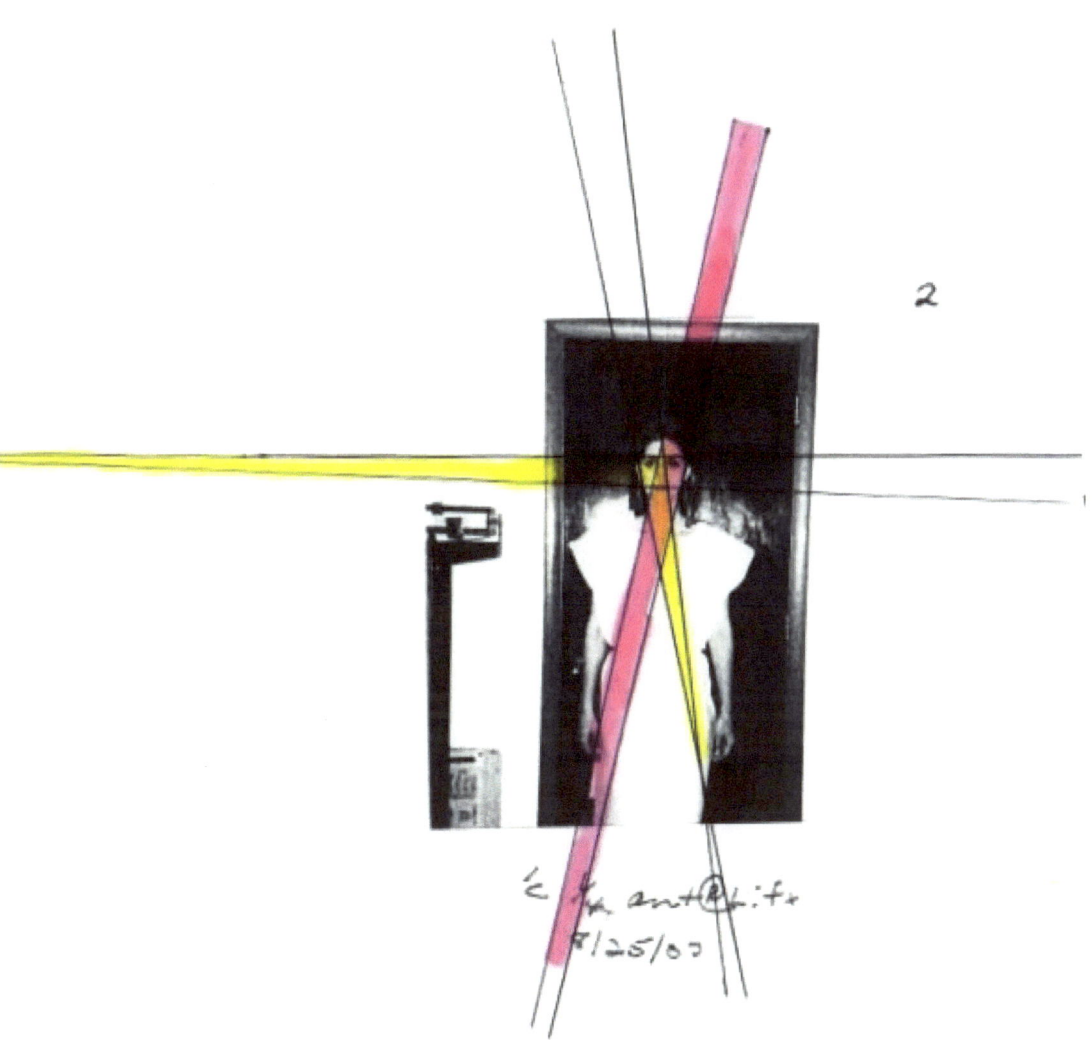

2

E.S.

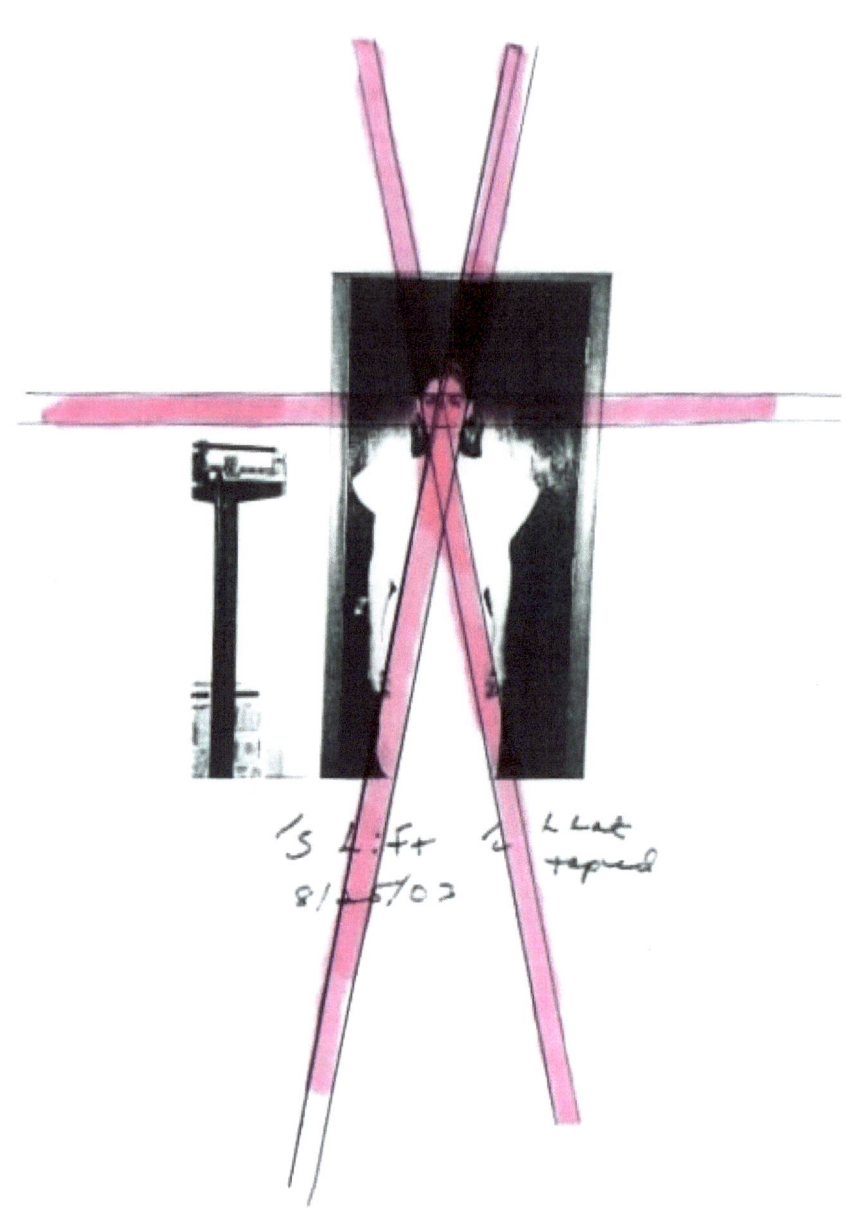

E.S.

08/25/03

She returns today. She is having a migraine about once every two weeks at this time. She feels that her neck has been cracking 20 to 30 times a day and sometime last semester she noted a change in her headaches. The patient notes 50 percent of the time when she cracks her neck her headache will leave. Diagnostic photography suggested she has bilateral internal rotation. I note that she has a little scoliosis today. She has not been wearing her lift for a while because she lost it. I did digital rectal examination to release the subluxation of the left coccyx cornua. I taped the lateral left foot to offset the posterior strain. I then did total mobilization of the craniosacral, visceral and musculoskeletal including the hands, feet and elbows. Posttreatment photograph with the lateral foot taped shows the patient to be symmetrical in three dimensions. She felt like she was going to have a migraine tomorrow and I suspect that we have aborted that at this time.   JAC:pb

96

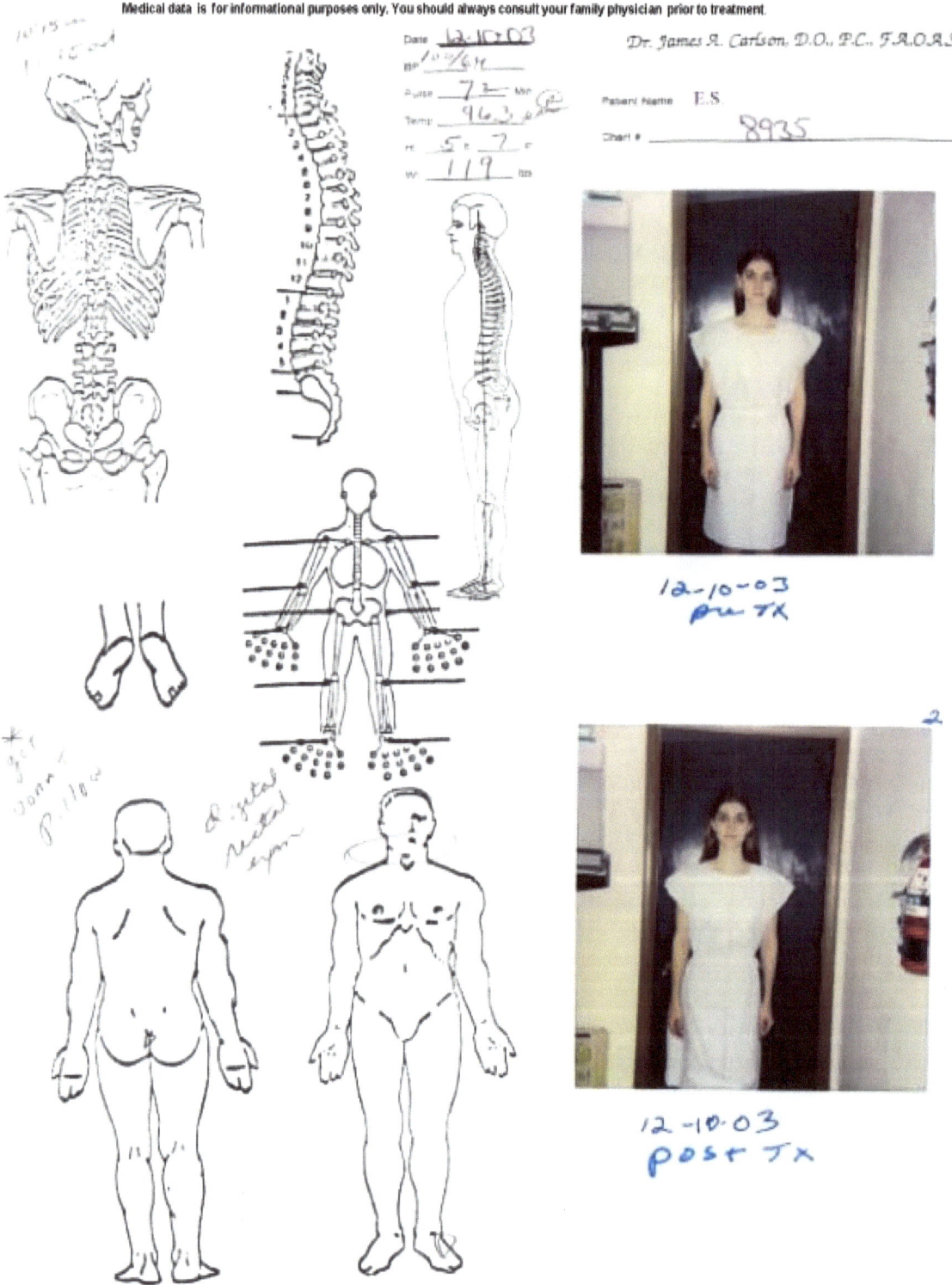

Date 12-10-03

Dr. James A. Carlson, D.O., P.C., F.A.O.A.S.

BP 112/64

Pulse 72 Min

Patient Name E.S

Temp 96.3

Chart # 8935

H 5' 7"

W 119 lbs

12-10-03
pre TX

2

12-10-03
post TX

97

Dr. James A. Carlson D.O., F.A.O.A.S.

Knoxville, Tennessee 37923
Musculo · Skeletal & Athletic Medicine

Patient E.S.   Chart # 8935   Page

Date 12-10-03 Progress   Plans

Subj.............................

H 'As are bad

Hurlchny approx 3 mbr ago
& full load pop H 'A's were
the worse

XXX..........................

Discussed i pt re: coccyx
Pt will discuss c her
mother re: lig. on coccix (coccyx
poss needs an xy i that area

X-Ray & Thermography......

Lab............................

Diagnostic Photos..............

Tx............................

Dx............................

Future Plans.......................
Status................................

Plans:
① omg Comp: Ca/mee
② spec. al crani al
    tech: Cas/mee
③ Diag Photos
④ digital contal sen

Pt is to return prn

E.S

2

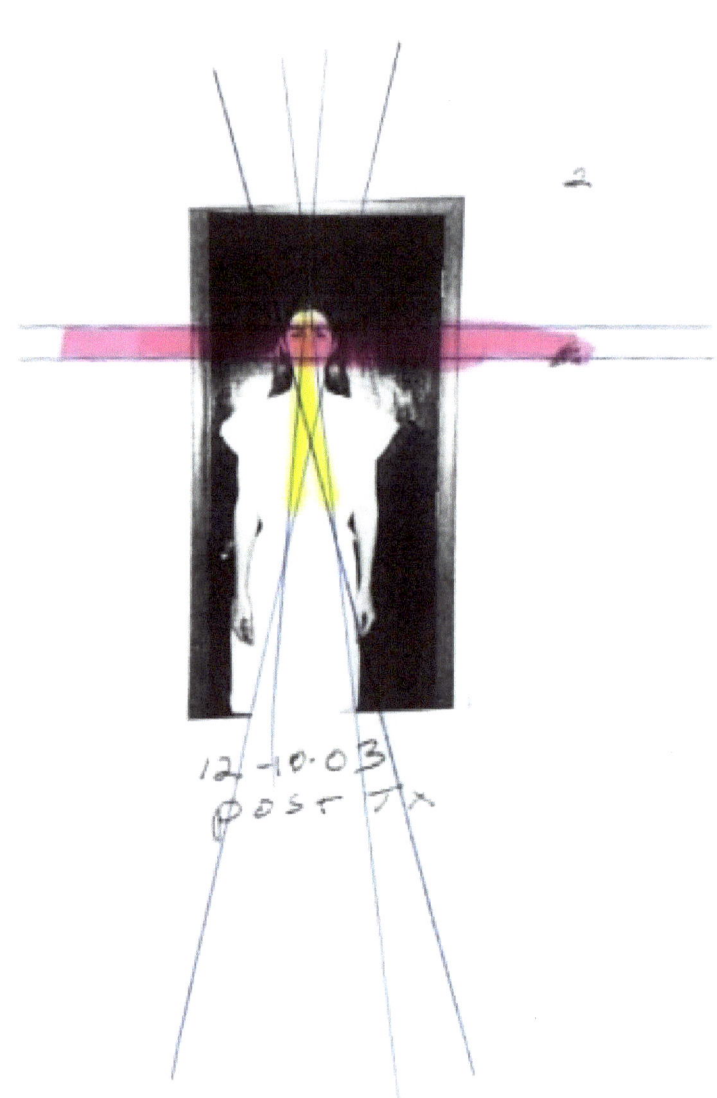

12-10-03
POST TX

99

F.S.

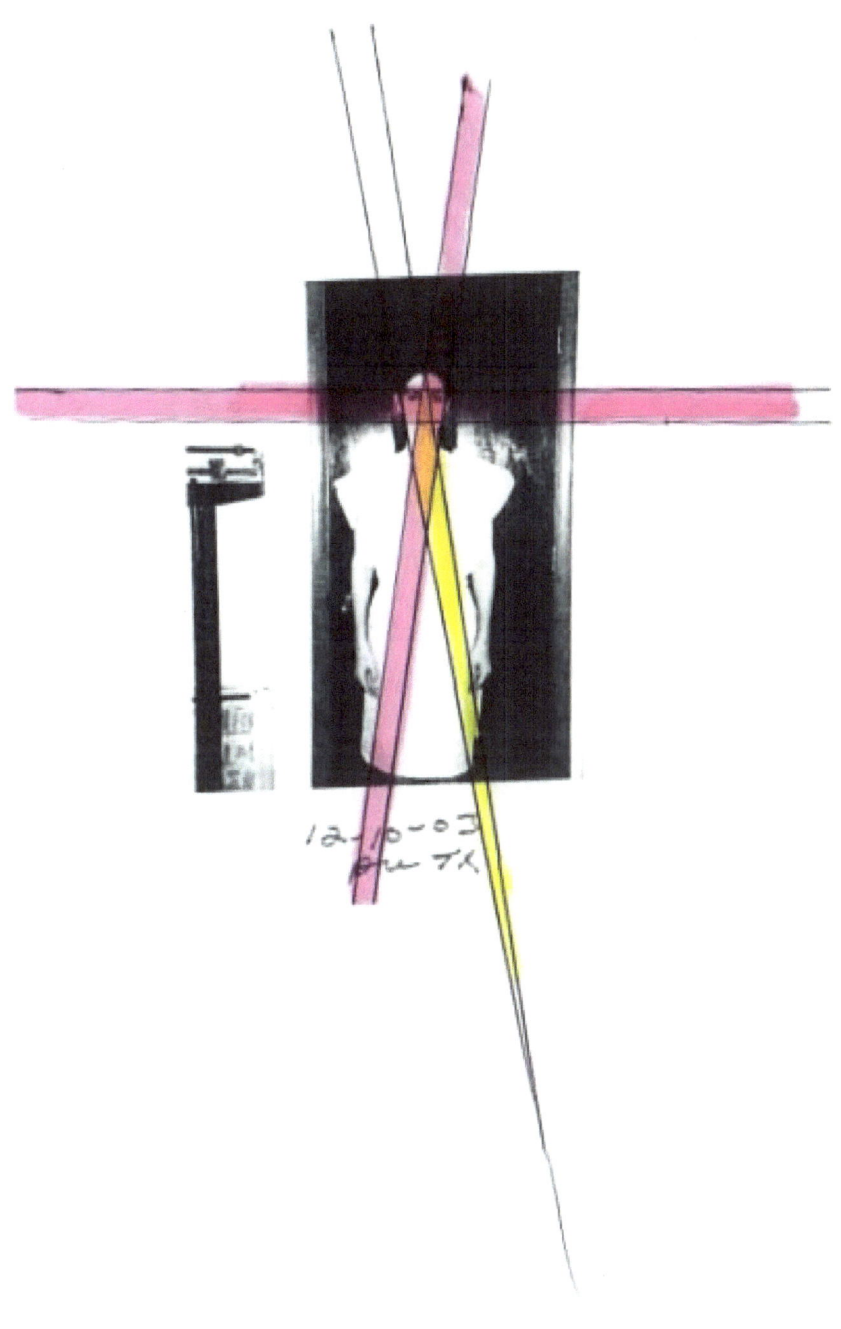

E.S.

12/10/03

She returns. She is just about through with final exams and she is going home to Maryland. She has had increasing headaches again. She says she shook them off and then by doing some stretches and felt a pop in her lower back and then it seemed that this started them and I think that it was her coccyx that was subluxed to the left. She also had cuboid and Achilles tendon involvement on the left with tenderness of the Achilles tendon and a sciatic pattern. This shows on her photograph. Total mobilization was done of the craniosacral, visceral and musculoskeletal. We did cranial mobilization but follow-up picture showed that she still had bilateral internal rotation so we did digital dactylization of the nasion which corrected her marked problem there and I feel that she will probably do fairly well now. I asked her to return before her next exams or p.r.n. I have also given her the name of Steve _____ in Arlington, Virginia for her little brother to see. Apparently he fractured his jaw some years ago in a bicycle accident and they are about to do surgery and she wanted somebody to evaluate him before the surgery and I think Steve would be the ideal person for them to see.   JAC:pb

101

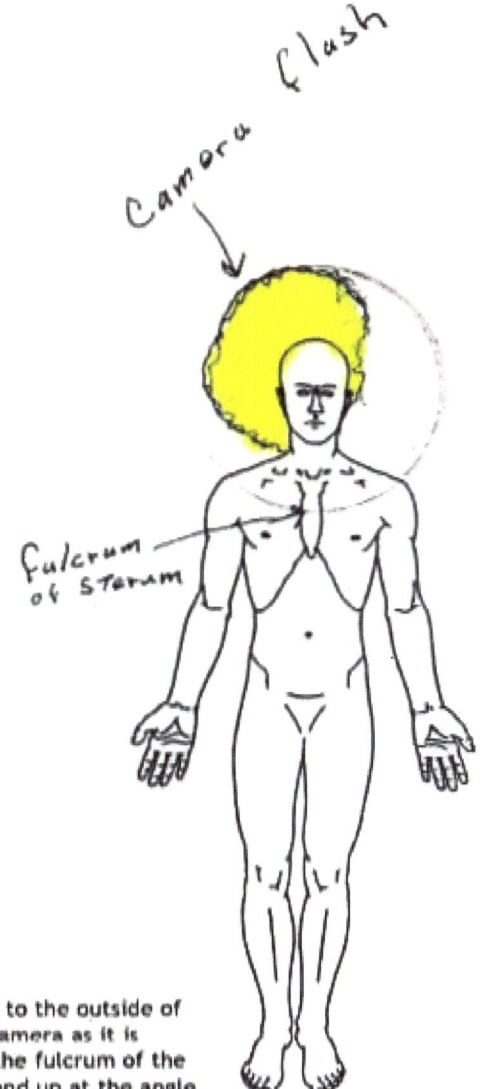

FIGURE 22.

The diameter between the eyes to the outside of
the flash on the wall from the camera as it is
brought around will determine the fulcrum of the
sternum. A normal flash would end up at the angle
of Louie which is normal fulcrum.

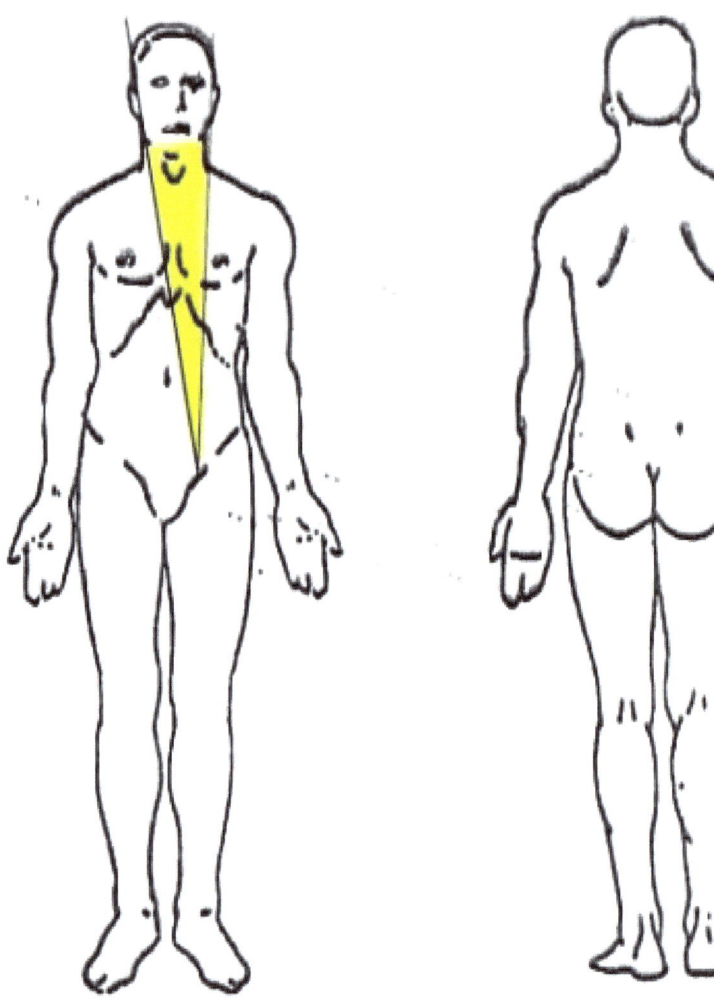

Prostate or Obturator Lo Inguinal
same side

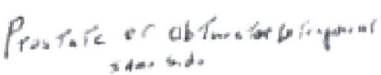

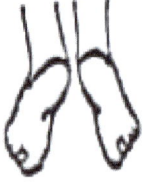
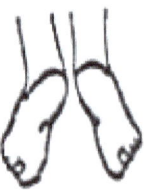

When this pattern occurs, it's almost always
a prostate problem on the side of the pattern.

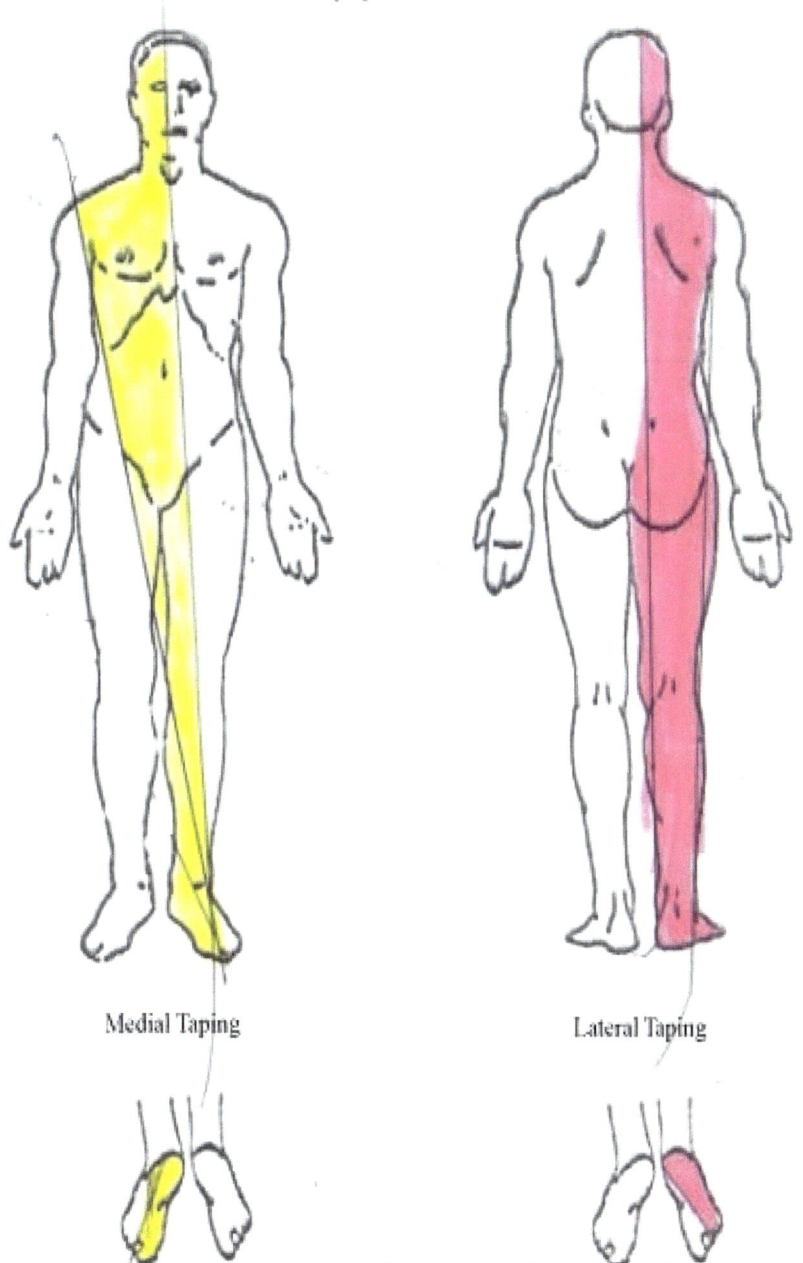

Medial Taping   Lateral Taping

The right pattern is an internal inhalation and parasympathetic pattern.
The anterior vector is flexion, inhalation and sympathetic and creates rotation.
Combination of these two patterns create torsion.

INSTRUCTIONS

1. When you have made photos of your patient, draw stress vectors on the pictures.

2. Apply tape to the patient's feet to counter the stress vectors, as per the following pictures.

3. This is a system that is particularly helpful as a two-person cranial mobilization technique. Two person cranial mobilization can be performed with the operator at the head of the table palpating the head for cranial disfunction. The assistant applies forward pressure to the taped feet as the operator continues and finishes the mobilization.

4. Following manipulation, the tape should be left on for 2 to 3 days to allow the body to continue its unwinding process.

5. The patient can shower, but baths will intefere with the strength of the taping.

6. The patient must walk, and also the patient should drink copious amounts of water.

7. The tape can be removed after 2 to 3 days.

Lateral Taping -- Step 1

Lateral Taping -- Step 2

Lateral Taping -- Step 3

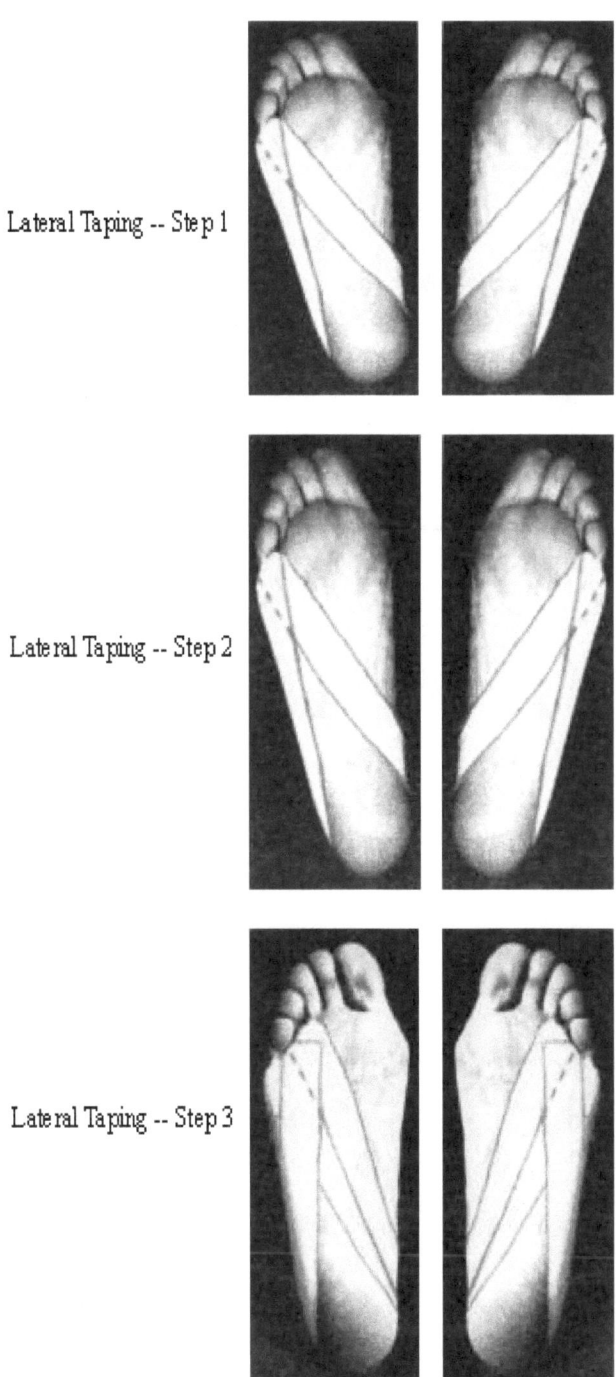

Use one inch Johnson & Johnson Zonas Porous Athletic Trainer's Tape.
If the foot is sweaty, you may have to first apply Tuff Skin spray. If the
skin is dry, then apply the Zonas tape directly.

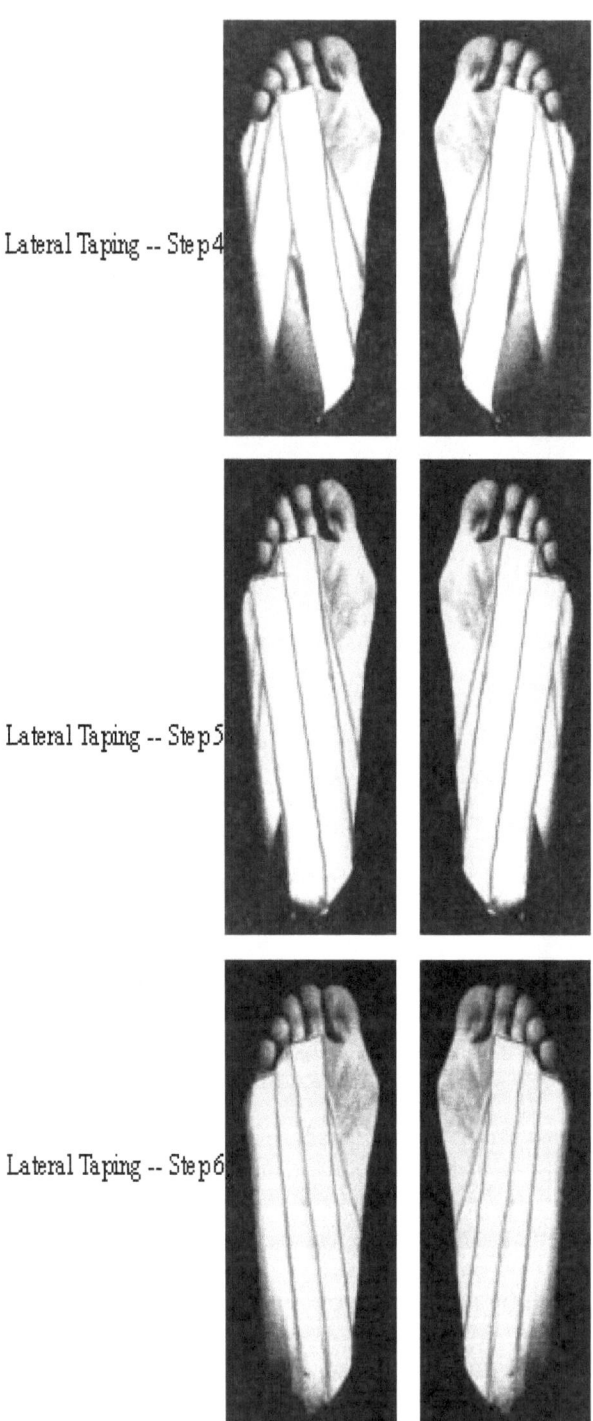

Lateral Taping -- Step 4

Lateral Taping -- Step 5

Lateral Taping -- Step 6

Medial Taping -- Step 1

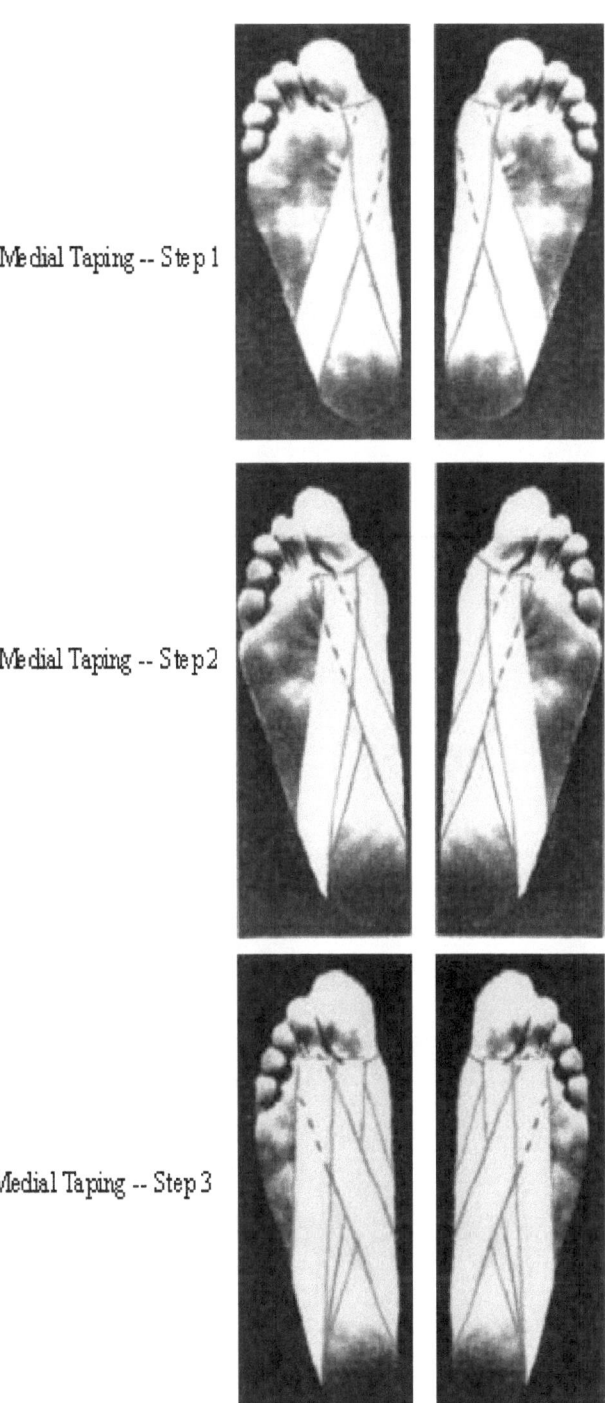

Medial Taping -- Step 2

Medial Taping -- Step 3

Medial Taping -- Step 4

Medial Taping -- Step 5

Medial Taping -- Step 6

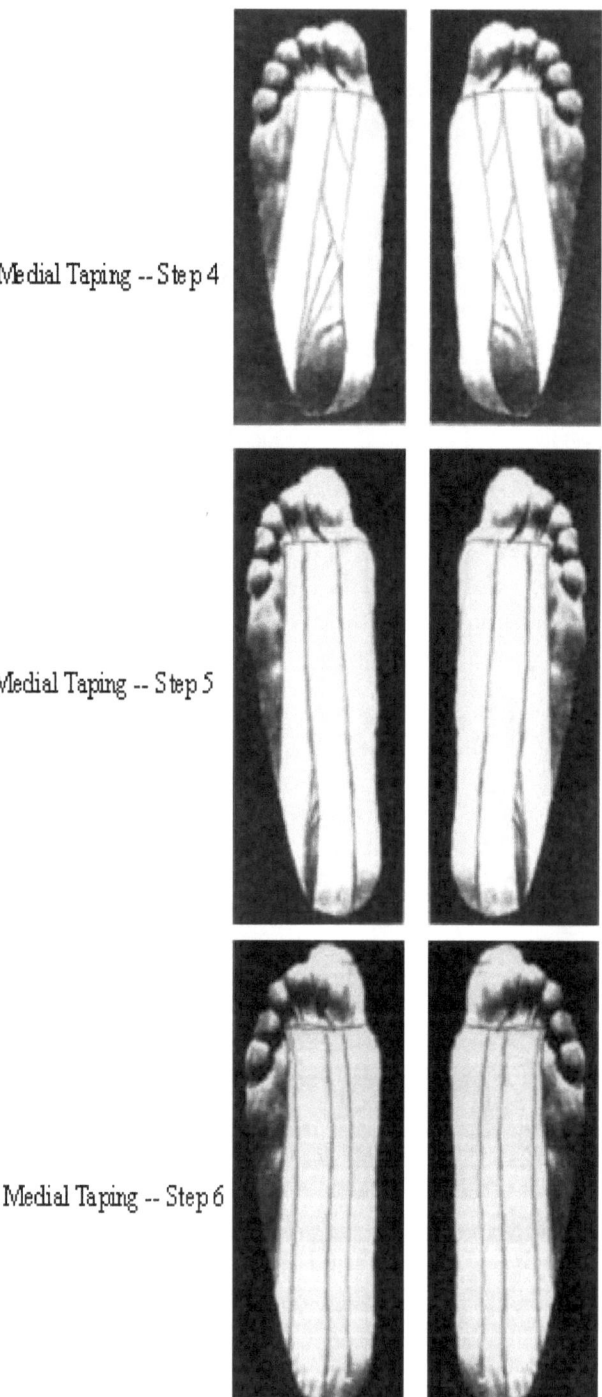

Total Taping -- Step 1

Total Taping -- Step 2

Total Taping -- Step 3

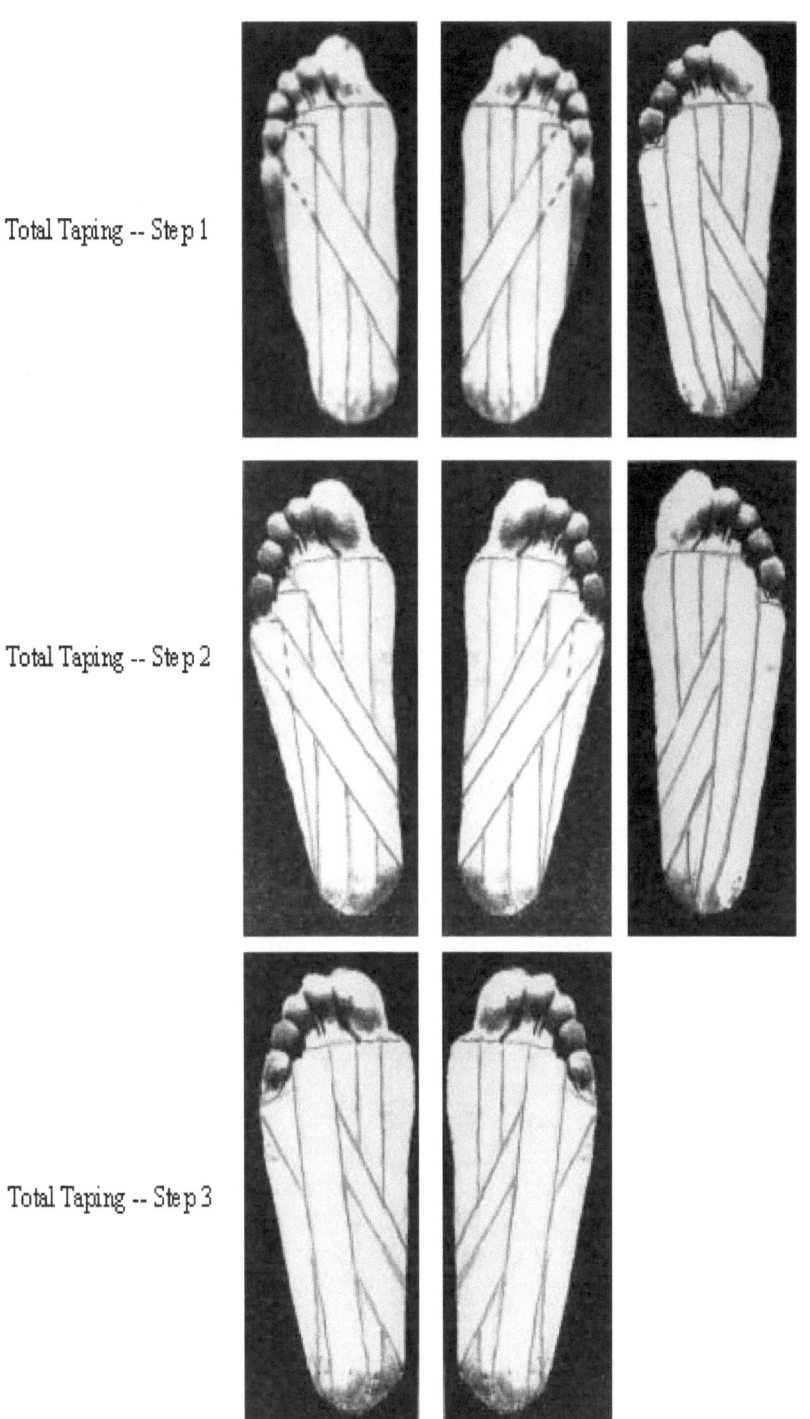

In Memoriam:
James Carlson, D.O.

✝✝ December 3, 1933 📖📖 July 3, 2011 ✝✝

by Perry A.Chapdelaine,Sr.

The Roger Wyburn-Mason and Jack M. Blount Foundation

for the Eradication of Rheumatoid Disease

aka The Arthritis Trust of America/

The Rheumatoid Disease Foundation

Every generation looks back on those they consider pioneers -- the "old timers."

The medical field of reconstructive therapy, or "prolo" therapy is no different. New practitioners of this field -- of which there are altogether too few -- have looked back to Jim Carlson, D.O. as one of the early pioneers.

Just last month my wife visited a beginning practitioner who thanked us for giving him a copy of "the old timer's" -- Carlson's -- work entitled *Structural Diagnostic Photography.*

Jim had been studying a new method of determining which tendons or ligaments needed attention. Although I'd known Jim and his wife, Brenda, for many years, and he was at first my osteopathic physician and then my close friend, I never saw him so enthusiastic as when he'd decided, at last, that his new system worked. It was elegantly simple. I offered out of friendship to computer lay-out a booklet for him.

In his turn he was kind enough to permit The Arthritis Trust of America to make it available first through our website at http:// www.arthritistrust.org and then later on through the website to Amazon.Com at kindle or directly, in book form, from Amazon.com at a very low cost.

Pre-med students usually study anatomy in their Freshman year. By the time they graduate and start administering to sick people -- except for certain medical specialties -- much of their gross memorization of Latin words has escaped them. Jim's knowledge of human anatomy was exceptional! In fact, I often accused him of being able to speak only in a dead language, such was his detailed memory of the names of parts of the human body.

Carlson knew the names of every little tidbit or bump in the body -- but most importantly he knew how everything affected everything else. He'd trot out anatomy charts and graphs and books and -- speaking their specialized medical language -- Jim would explain how this part of the body acted as a fulcrum and another as a lever, how this part acted like a pulley belt and this part as a pulley wheel.

When he was through with his explanations the patient would understand why Jim would be treating a portion of the body far removed from the pain. When I'd shrug off the medical words, at last, in English, he'd say, "I have to treat this part here because it connects to this part and that affects this part and that affects this part . . . ." It always reminded me of the old song where the skull bone finally gets connected to the anklebone!

When I first met Jim I was suffering terribly day and night with shoulder/neck pain. Traditional osteopaths wanted to operate, but they could never explain why, or whether or not I'd be pain free. Even if so, would I still have my range of motion?

Dr. Faber, prolo therapist from Wisconsin, referred me to Dr. Carlson. I began seeing Carlson once a month. It took eleven months, eleven treatments, whence I was totally pain free. I've been so now for more than a quarter of a century.

Why did it take so long?

I lived a seven hour round trip drive away and my income at the time was very low. More importantly, my metabolism was low. Effectiveness of reconstructive therapy depends upon the rate at which one can heal oneself and that, in turn, depends on one's metabolism. Jim said that I would have responded in several weeks with a higher metabolism and more frequent treatments.

I used to dance jitterbug style 365 days a week into my seventies. A friend I'd sent to Carlson for treatment told them about the number of beautiful girls this old codger always had at his table. When my turn for a patient visit arrived Jim and his wife, Brenda, asked me about this unusual statement. I was lying on his treatment table with only a pair of shorts, my aging body exposed and available for his multitude of needles.

I said, "Folks, they're not interested in me, just in using my body."

They each took one look at my aging frame and broke out in virtually uncontrollable gales of laughter.

The beautiful girls were, of course, interested in my dancing skill, not this aging frame.

I was greatly impressed with Jim Carlson at the very first. I'd never before met a doctor who would spend anywhere from one to three hours with each patient. Most today warehouse one in a small room, have his nurse take vitals, then, after a boring wait, the doctor will bounce in to ask a few questions. He'll quickly write a prescription and then charge out to the next little cubicle.

Not Jim!

When he accepted a patient he gave them his full attention, using every device he had to make his diagnosis and corrections.

Little by little, as our friendship grew, I noted that he discarded first one device or test or another until he was left with a Polaroid camera, a plumb bob on a string, a pencil and straight edge. These at last became his primary diagnostic tools outside of his fascinating knowledge of anatomy. His methods were finally made available to other doctors through this book, *A New Diagnostic Tool for Prolo Therapy: Structural Diagnostic Photography.*

Do not think that he arrived at this diagnostic short cut willy-nilly. Years passed in their testing and trials before he finally accepted the validity of these new ideas.

He'd take a Polaroid picture of his patient standing behind the plumb bob on a string in a standardized position. Then he'd retire to his office with the picture where he'd use the straight edge and colored pencils to draw lines connecting stress indicators everywhere seen on the body: face, shoulders, legs, etc.

Depending upon the nature and geometry of the interaction of these stress lines would determine where he'd search for treatment needs.

The whole was indeed brilliant, simple, yes, even elegant!

From time to time I'd visit Brenda and Jim and once they came to my house to stay for a month.

I truly enjoyed their company!

As soon as I returned home from a year's absence in the Philippines I visited my old friends in Knoxville, finding Jim unable to walk but otherwise still bright and -- may I say it? -- lovable.

I'm so glad that I got to visit one last time before he peacefully passed on.